THE WAGES OF SEEKING HELP

THE WAGES OF SEEKING HELP

Sexual Exploitation by Professionals

CAROL BOHMER

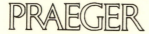

Westport, Connecticut
London

Library of Congress Cataloging-in-Publication Data

Bohmer, Carol.
   The wages of seeking help : sexual exploitation by professionals / Carol Bohmer.
      p. cm.
   Includes bibliographical references and index.
   ISBN 0–275–96793–X (alk. paper)
      1. Sexually abused patients.   2. Medical personnel and patient.   3. Medical
   personnel—Sexual behavior.   4. Sexual abuse victims.   I. Title.
   RC560.S44 B67 2000
      616.85´83—dc21   99–045991

British Library Cataloguing in Publication Data is available.

Library of Congress Catalog Card Number: 99–045991
ISBN: 0–275–96793–X

First published in 2000

Praeger Publishers, 88 Post Road West, Westport, CT 06881
An imprint of Greenwood Publishing Group, Inc.
www.praeger.com

Printed in the United States of America

The paper used in this book complies with the
Permanent Paper Standard issued by the National
Information Standards Organization (Z39.48-1984).

10 9 8 7 6 5 4 3 2 1

Copyright Acknowledgments

Portions of Chapter 3 were previously published as "Victims Who Fight Back: Claiming in Cases of Professional Sexual Exploitation," *Justice System Journal* 16.3 (1994): 73–92, and are reprinted with permission of the publisher.

Portions of Chapter 4 were previously published as "Failure and Success in Self-Help Groups for Victims of Professional Sexual Exploitation," *Journal of Community Psychology* (July 1995): 190–199.

Every reasonable effort has been made to trace the owners of copyright materials in this book, but in some instances this has proven impossible. The author and publisher will be glad to receive information leading to more complete acknowledgments in subsequent printings of the book and in the meantime extend their apologies for any omissions.

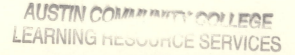

*To the memory
of
my father*

CONTENTS

ACKNOWLEDGMENTS

I would like to thank all the people who helped me in the several years it took to write this book. Special thanks go to the students who provided research: Else Slepecky, Lauren Weldon, Gail McGuire, Valerie Rake, and Jelena Batinic were all of great assistance. It is impossible to name all those who gave so freely of their time and effort, but Gary Schoener deserves to be singled out for the patience and enthusiasm with which he answered my many questions over the years. Many other professionals gave generously of their time, for which I am immensely grateful. Those many people who were exploited by professionals and who made the effort to tell me of their usually painful experiences provided me with invaluable material. Without their courage and willingness to share, this book could not have been written.

I would like to thank my family for their support, and those friends who encouraged me to keep going. You know who you are.

I would also like to acknowledge the Graduate School of Public and International Affairs, University of Pittsburgh, and Ohio State University for the research support they provided me.

— 1 —

INTRODUCTION

"Tangled Case of Sexual Molestation Pits a Doctor against 8 Poor Women"

—Lewin, 1995

"Psychiatrists and Sex Abuse: State Regulation Marked by Delay, Confusion, Loopholes"

—Lehr, 1994

The last couple of decades have brought to public attention several issues of violence and exploitation against women. Domestic violence and rape have attracted the most attention, both from feminists and, more recently, from the general public. But other problems with women as their primary victims have not received much public attention.

Professional sexual misconduct (also called exploitation or abuse) is such an issue. Over the last few years we have learned that all professional relationships are not always the source of comfort and help they have been held out to be. For some, it appears that the cure may be worse than the disease. A patient who gets involved in a sexual relationship with her therapist "for her benefit" finds that the benefit was all for the therapist. An emotionally distraught divorce client receives demands for payment in sex as well as money for her lawyer's services. A woman goes to a clergyman for pastoral counseling and gets propositioned. A gynecological exam becomes the occasion for a doctor's sexual gratification.

Incidence studies have shown that 4–13 percent of all therapists engage in sexual contact with their patients, while the figure for lawyers is 7 percent (Schoener, 1989b; Murrell et al., 1993), and one estimate of priests puts the figure at 5–10 percent (Greeley, 1993). Approximately 80 percent of the perpetrators are male and the victims female, and a large number of the perpetrators are repeaters (Bouhoutsos et al., 1983; Holroyd and Brodsky, 1977; Gartrell et al., 1986).

There are a couple of reasons that this is a problem whose victims are primarily women. Despite inroads by women into the professions, more professionals are still male and therefore potential exploiters. In addition, women are more inclined to seek the help of professionals, especially medical and therapeutic professionals.

We as a society are ambivalent about seeking help. We believe that it is OK to make efforts to help oneself in times of difficulty, as witness the legions of self-help books on the shelves of bookstores. It is also OK to seek out others who are suffering from the same difficulty, as we can see from the church basements and other public spaces that are packed with support groups for every conceivable problem, as well as their cyberspace counterparts, Internet chat-rooms.

What is much less OK is to seek out therapeutic help. When it is revealed that a public figure, especially a politician, has sought psychiatric help, the result is punishment or, at best, a lack of understanding for his or her "weakness." While this reaction seems, at present, to be stronger against men, that may be simply because fewer women are political figures. Nevertheless, it typifies public attitudes toward help-seeking behavior for "mental" problems.

The help-seeking aspect of this problem and society's reaction to it are central to an understanding of how professional sexual misconduct is framed and perceived by the public. Women are not the only victims of the behavior; nor is it by any means confined to therapists. However, social attitudes and bureaucratic responses are tainted by our views of therapy and of women who seek help. Women who are sexually exploited by professionals are twice punished. The first time they are punished for having sought help and having thus "asked for" the sexual behavior. They are punished a second time in their efforts to claim redress for the exploitation. For many, the process of obtaining redress is too arduous or traumatic even to undertake it; those who do make a public claim find themselves engaged in a long, unpleasant experience with major financial and emotional costs.

The literature on rape and domestic violence is replete with evidence that blaming the victim is commonplace, especially when the issue of consent is in question, as in acquaintance rape. These punitive attitudes seem to have softened a bit lately in the case of domestic violence and rape. Mandatory arrest of batterers and the passage in 1994 of the Violence Against Women Act are two examples of the increasing recognition of the legitimacy of domestic violence and rape as social problems.

Despite the increased public attention to these other issues affecting women, it is apparent that professional sexual exploitation must go through the same process of obtaining recognition by the public as well as those directly concerned with the issue. Claims-makers have also had to respond to arguments that this is a private issue of consensual sex, without the evidence of violence that can negate claims of having "asked for it" or "wanted it," as is more often the case in battering and rape. Embedded in these arguments is our society's profound ambivalence about sex and our complex and often contradictory attitudes toward appropriate female behavior.

So far, claims-makers have not been very successful in gaining public recognition for professional sexual exploitation. Most people have never even heard the term and do not know what it means. Nor have efforts to initiate social change from either the public or the relevant professional community had more than mixed success. One of the foci of this book is to examine the reasons this is so.

The rhetoric of power and dominance has been an important element in the discourse of the women's movement, and it is particularly important in an explanation of the history and construction of professional sexual misconduct. It also illustrates the connections between professional sexual misconduct and other problems primarily affecting women as well as differences among the problems.

Power is central to the construction of professional sexual exploitation on three different levels. At one level, since we are speaking of a claim most often made by a woman against a man, there is the power inherent in that relationship. At a second level, doctors, lawyers, and the clergy (the professionals most frequently accused) are among the highest-status members of our society. At a third level, allegations of professional sexual exploitation are sometimes made against men who hold social power within their profession in addition to the power generated by their gender and their profession (Noel with Watterson, 1992; Walker and Young, 1986). These three levels at which power is central distinguish professional sexual exploitation from other social problems in which female victims predominate. For example, most perpetrators of rape are not particularly powerful individuals themselves and therefore have the protection only of their gender, rather than their gender and their social position of power.

The social roles of a person in need of help and a person providing that help exacerbate the power imbalance, especially when the patient or client is female. In fact, the fatherly professional responding to the needs of the childlike patient or client is the archetypical patriarchal relationship. It can be argued that the power imbalance is inherent in the relationship rather than in the gender of the respective participants in it, though its source is the classic patriarchal power relationship of male professional and female patient or client. Thus, the power imbalance survives the entrance of women into the professions under discussion.

Like the construction of other social problems, those framing the problem are both professionals who deal with it in their work and victims themselves. But in this case the very people who would, in other social problems, be among the claims-makers (the professionals) are themselves the "cause" of the "problem." This leads to divisions within the professions because members of the professions are particularly needed in constructing the problem to provide "expert" status and, in addition, to enhance the credibility of the claims. But when professionals do lend status and credibility in the construction of the social problem, they are thereby required to criticize their colleagues, something many professionals are reluctant to do. By contrast, professionals constructing other social problems are not caught in this bind. For example, child abuse was originally constructed by a small group of doctors who publicized the need for their colleagues to recognize the signs of abuse in their patients that they had previously ignored (Nelson, 1984). In that case, the doctors were encouraged to become involved in exposing the problem, not accused of causing it.

Because the issue of psychological harm is a central element of the claim, professionals are needed even more than they are in the case of some other problems, like child abuse and even woman-battering and stranger rape, because in those cases at least some components of the trauma are visible. In cases of nonviolent professional sexual exploitation, the problem needs to be framed in ways that stress the harm caused; otherwise, it will simply be seen (as it may be anyway) as just a romantic relationship between professional and client/patient. Even in the case of sexual harassment, in which the relationship may be viewed as an ordinary sexual encounter, claimants can often provide externally verifiable evidence such as being fired from a job or failing a course in which the victim had previously been doing well. The case of hostile environment sexual harassment (where the creation of a sexually offensive atmosphere is central to the claim) is more similar to that of professional sexual exploitation. Outsiders may not "get" why the victim felt she had to leave the job or the school when the damage on which she bases her claim is less tangible. This is even clearer in the case of professional sexual misconduct. Since the victim was already in need of professional help, she is defined, at best, as "troubled" and, at worst, as "crazy." The negative effect of professional sexual exploitation on her psychological condition can usually be fully measured only by another professional.

Many claims-makers in professional sexual exploitation, including professionals, are themselves victims of professional sexual abuse and, therefore, mostly women. Because women have a lower status in the professions than their male counterparts in general, female professionals have a hard time being taken seriously in their efforts to frame the social problem. As we have seen, most of the professionals who engage in professional sexual exploitation are men. So are the most powerful members of the professional organizations. For the most part, women are marginal in their professional organizations. Thus, when a woman professional expresses her concern about the existence and extent of the problem, she has less credibility than her male counterparts and risks further marginalization in the organization.

The experience of Nanette Gartrell and her female colleagues (1987) in trying to get the American Psychiatric Association (APA) to conduct an incidence study of sexual exploitation among psychiatrists provides a telling illustration of the difficulties involved in persuading male-dominated professional organizations to address the problem. They recount extensive resistance on the part of the APA to respond to the call by the Committee on Women of the APA to undertake the study. Two years of efforts by the Committee on Women failed to persuade the APA to sponsor the survey, so the study was ultimately conducted independently.

A SHORT HISTORY OF PROFESSIONAL
SEXUAL MISCONDUCT

Professional sexual exploitation has been the subject of regulation since it was first mentioned in the Hippocratic oath in about the fourth or fifth century B.C. (Schoener, 1995). The relevant part of the oath reads: "In every house where I come I will enter only for the good of my patients, keeping myself far from all intentional ill-doing and all seduction, and especially from the pleasures of love with women or with men, be they free or slaves" (*Stedman's Medical Dictionary*, 1990: 716–17).

Despite this ancient and respectable origin, until recently, sexual exploitation by professionals of their clients and patients was abhorred by some, accepted as therapeutic by a few, and unacknowledged by most. In recent years, however, the subject has become one of professional concern and has received some publicity in the media. In fact, many claims-makers have used its long history of neglect as a rallying cry for activism: "[T]wenty-four centuries are enough," they say (Schoener, 1995).

The issue became more focused with the development of Freudian psychology. This had to do with its emphasis on the relationship between therapist and patient, its description of the concept of transference, and the apparent evidence that Freud and his colleagues themselves seem to have had various forms of sexual relationships with their patients.

Freud provided an intellectual/therapeutic framework for the construction of the behavior as a social problem by his discussion of the phenomenon of transference. He pointed out that his female patients had romantic and erotic feelings toward him (Freud, 1958). According to psychoanalytic theory, these feelings are transferred from someone in the patient's past onto the therapist. Likewise, the therapist brings to the relationship his own set of feelings (known as countertransference), which come from his own early experience as well as in response to the patient's feelings for

him. Thus, these feelings on the part of both therapist and patient are connected to the therapeutic process and are not the same as feelings that exist in ordinary relationships. For this reason, a therapist who engages in a
sexual relationship with a patient is taking advantage of a phenomenon
caused by the therapy itself, which can greatly interfere with any benefits
of the therapy. Despite Freud's warnings against it, some of his colleagues
and followers (including Ferenczi, Jung, and Horney) did experiment with
physical contact with patients (Schoener, 1989b).

The issue was not raised as an ethical dilemma for therapists but rather
as a complicating feature of treatment. With the emphasis on transference,
it is possible to see the "problem" as a manifestation of the patient's illness rather than as inappropriate behavior on the part of the therapist
(Davidson, 1977). Professional sexual exploitation occurs when the therapist acts on the feelings of "love" the patient exhibits for him as if they
were real, rather than part of the therapeutic process. The use of sex by
doctors as a medical procedure for their patients has had a checkered, if
little known, history. Late in the last century, doctors were provided with
a mechanical device to relieve tension in their female patients: the vibrator (Maines, 1999). This device was a substitute for a service they were apparently already providing manually as a way of dealing with what
Freud and others considered a major disease of women: hysteria or
"neurasthenia." For the doctors, we are told, this was not a matter of their
own sexual pleasure but something they did "because they felt it was
their duty" (Angier, 1999).

Ironically, professional sexual misconduct was most recently framed as
a social problem as a result of the popularity of various trendy forms of
therapy of the touchy-feely kind in the 1960s and 1970s. The human potential movement, which included encounter groups and alternative therapy, among other things, blurred the lines between therapist and patient.
As part of that movement, there was some debate in the profession, with
a few voices arguing that sexual contact between patient and therapist
might be therapeutically helpful or at least should be studied in an un-
biased manner (McCartney, 1966; Shepard, 1971). These claims of acceptability by even fringe members of the profession gave great impetus to
those constructing professional sexual exploitation as a social problem.
The strength of the backlash against the suggestion that patient–therapist
sex might have a place in therapy is illustrated by the inability of a psychiatrist named Clay Dahlberg to get an article (which did no more than
advocate further study) published in the professional journals. Dahlberg's
article described cases of which he had clinical knowledge in which he argued that the effect of therapist–patient sex ranged from "relatively harm-
less" to "frankly destructive" (Dahlberg, 1970: 107, 111). He was in no way
endorsing the practice, merely its study, but nevertheless, no journal
would publish his article. Some of the backlash might also have been the

result of a need on the part of mainstream therapy to distance itself from the "new" therapies that were springing up all over and gaining more acceptance than the traditionalists wanted. McCartney and Shepard were both ultimately expelled from the profession, though Shepard denied that he himself had engaged in sexual relations with his patients.

The development of sex therapy and the use of sexual surrogates also contributed to the idea that therapist–patient sex might have positive benefits. As long as the therapy is about improving the sexual functioning of a patient, it is very difficult to delineate clearly the line between therapy and sex. The use of sex surrogates is important here; it raises the specter of a therapist's "pimping" for his patient, while any sex therapy that the therapist does himself has overtones of exploitation.

Masters and Johnson, who pioneered the treatment of sexual dysfunction, spoke out very early against sexual relationships between therapist and patient (Masters and Johnson, 1970: 388–91; 1975). In fact, their discussion of the subject in their 1970 book appears to be the first time it was suggested that therapist–patient sex was not limited to those who could be dismissed as pseudotherapists. However, it took a long time after this for the profession to come out publicly and denounce professional exploitation, as well as to admit how widespread it was.

In the late 1970s and early 1980s, the momentum against professional sexual misconduct began to build both in the profession and among the general public. One of the major triggers for this concern was the publication of a book by Julie Roy, who described her sexual exploitation at the hands of her psychiatrist (Freeman and Roy, 1976). In 1985 Seymour Zelen said that "(s)exual abuse of patients has come out of the closet" (Zelen, 1985). This public attention also coincided with the dissemination of a number of incidence studies that provided claims-makers with ammunition on which to base their claim that the problem was widespread (Schoener, 1989b).

More recently, the social construction of professional sexual exploitation has been extended in two major ways. First, other professions in which there is a close professional–client relationship—from the clergy to lawyers, massage therapists to social workers—were included in the claims. The process has not, so far, succeeded in the case of lawyers. Many lawyers still believe that sex between client and lawyer is, at least some of the time, quite acceptable. In addition, there is a strong feeling that specific rules against sexual behavior violate attorneys' right to privacy and freedom of association (Firestone and Simon, 1992).

The second way in which the claims were extended was in the definition of the relationship. A therapist is now prohibited from engaging in sex with a patient even after therapy has terminated, though disagreement remains whether a sexual relationship is ever ethical with a former patient and if so, what the appropriate period is after the end of therapy (Lazarus,

1992). Current definitions of professional sexual misconduct (or exploitation or abuse) encompass sexual relationships (whether intercourse or other sexual activity, whether forced or not) in the professions. Definitions vary in their specificity depending on the purpose for which they are designed. For example, the American Psychiatric Association in its handbook on the principles of medical ethics says simply that "(s)exual activity with a current or former patient is unethical" (*The Principles of Medical Ethics*, 1993: 4). Some researchers use a broader definition in which professional sexual contact is defined as "behavior which is primarily intended to arouse or satisfy sexual desire" (Vinson, 1984: 30). In those states that have made sexual exploitation a criminal offense, the definition usually covers "(a)ny person who is or who holds himself or herself out to be a therapist and who intentionally has sexual contact with a patient or client during any ongoing therapist–patient or therapist–client relationship" (Wisc. Stat. Ann. s.940.22[2] 1990).

While inappropriate sexual contact takes place in other work-related settings, professional sexual exploitation is distinguished by the central element of confidentiality and trust in the relationship. Breach of confidentiality is an important element in the social construction of this problem. Inappropriate sexual behavior in other professional situations where confidentiality plays a smaller role, for example, professor and student or employer and employee, shares many features of professional sexual exploitation, especially the abuse of power. The legal remedies are different (and perhaps also the social and psychological ramifications), however, and it may be for this reason that this behavior has usually been constructed as sexual harassment rather than professional sexual exploitation.

THE SOCIAL MOVEMENT

Part of the explanation for professional sexual misconduct's relative lack of salience as a public issue lies in the lack of a social movement to put it on the public agenda. As a social movement, professional sexual misconduct is fragmented and not very well organized. Its activists number only in the few thousands and include primarily those people who have themselves been abused by a professional and a relatively small number of those with a professional interest in the issue. Those who have been abused by members of the clergy represent the most organized of the activists, and there are now several networks of varying levels of organization to cater to their needs. Those who have been exploited by therapists are less organized. There are some support groups in various parts of the country and one mostly local network. While these networks purport to represent all those who have been abused by professionals (and in some cases other victims also), there appears to be relatively little overlap between those abused by the clergy and those abused by therapists and other professionals. Not surprisingly, we shall see that these limitations of the movement have major ramifications for the "success" of the movement.

CONCLUSION

Despite its surface similarities to other issues of violence and exploitation against women, this problem seems to languish in the netherworld as an issue of great importance to a few but no importance to most. Most people outside the field do not know what the terms "professional sexual misconduct" or "professional sexual exploitation" mean. The support groups and organizations are not very successful and have not been able to attract a large membership or the interest of government agencies. No public figure has come forward as a spokesperson for the problem.

Subsequent chapters examine the construction of professional sexual misconduct as a social problem and explain some of the reasons for its lack of salience. The issue is tied into the current ambivalence in our society about sexual behavior, as well as about seeking help for psychological problems. Professional sexual exploitation is examined from the perspective of the individual victim, the organizations, and the legal system. The final chapter discusses what could be done to change the way it is framed and handled. Many of the insights are applicable in a broader context. They illustrate how women, sex, and help-seeking are perceived in our society in the 1990s.

—2—

FRAMING PROFESSIONAL
SEXUAL MISCONDUCT

[H]e said that he loved me. He said that he would help me to feel like
a woman. . . . I felt like it was part of my treatment. . . . I felt comfort
and solace. . . . I worshipped Dr. F____, and I felt he had all that was
good and that was healing.
                                        —A woman who had sex with her analyst.
                         Board of Registration in Medicine v. *Joel Feigen, M.D.*

INTRODUCTION

The meaning of social events is not self-evident; it assumes meaning
through social construction (Spector and Kitsuse, 1977). Social construction has enormous implications for an event's recognition as a social problem, that is, how it is perceived and what is done about it (Best, 1989,
1990). For an event to become a social problem in the eyes of the public
and those who would be in a position to "do something about it," it needs
to be framed in an appealing way. This chapter examines different ways in
which professional sexual exploitation is presented and the implications of
these various constructions for its social problem status. The quote that begins this chapter illustrates several possible frames of reference; sex between the therapist and his female patient was seen by her as treatment,
healing, solace (medical care), love (gender roles), and worship (power
relations).

There are two major sources for the frame of reference used to define
and respond to professional sexual exploitation: the women's movement
and the medical consumer movement. Frames that come directly out of
each of those movements cover only some aspects of what is seen as professional sexual exploitation (or misconduct or abuse). An expanded
frame being developed by activists in the field combines the two strands

of the problem and expands on it. It constructs the problem within a medical/professional/power framework that addresses gender indirectly by the use of power as a central element of that framework. Power can be seen here as both a proxy for gender and a means of including both male and female victims. This process is called domain expansion by social problem theorists (Best, 1990). As a mobilization technique, social movement theorists describe the process of aligning values and interests as frame extension and frame amplification (Snow et al., 1986).[1] It is a strategic process by social movements (or claims-makers) to position the issue more effectively in the public arena.

As we see in later chapters, efforts to construct an effective claim for the issue of professional sexual exploitation have not so far been very successful (see Snow and Benford, 1988; Snow et al., 1986). The issue has received only sporadic media attention. Efforts to change the law and public policy have had mixed success. Some states have passed special legislation to criminalize the behavior, but there have been very few prosecutions under the statutes and usually only in the most egregious cases (Noel, 1992; Bohmer, 1995b). Professional and regulatory organizations have made it clear that sexual behavior between a professional and a patient or client is inappropriate and a matter for their control. For the most part, however, such bodies are reluctant to take strong action (Bohmer, 1995b; Lehr, 1994). The issue appears to be one of low hierarchical salience for the potential audience (Snow et al., 1986). It is considered insufficiently serious in contrast to other, related issues that are seen as "much worse," like medical malpractice and violent crime, which cause physical, rather than psychological, harm.

Johnson et al. (1994) argue that "status movements take action about 'other people's business' because that business often poses a threat to how the mobilizing group defines itself" (23). Professional sexual misconduct is not at present seen as a threat to the various potential mobilizing groups (feminists, medical consumers, and religious groups). McCarthy (1994) points out that "a frame must resonate with the experience of a collectivity and be accessible with its mix of crosscutting identities" (134). Relatively few people, however, see themselves as potential patients or clients in the mental health setting, and many members of religious congregations see clergy abuse as something that happens to children and in other denominations. So the problem of professional sexual misconduct remains "other people's business," of importance only to those who have suffered because of it. Seeking help is, in general, viewed as an expression of weakness and therefore something many people have no wish to identify with. As one writer puts it: "Although educated people may support the idea of therapy in public, in reality the stigma associated with seeking therapy remains culturally entrenched" (Pagano, 1997b).

The problem of defining professional sexual misconduct is compounded by the limitations of the different frames. If it is framed as a feminist issue, then it is definitely "other people's business" to those for whom it is a medical or a religious issue. The same is, of course, true in reverse. The expanded frame I describe here has the potential to be more robust because it is linked to a wider variety of values (Snow and Benford, 1988). It also has the advantage of connecting the various different strands of the movement to include sexual abuse in the medical context and by the clergy and other professionals. It may be more effective in generating sustained public interest, which will lead to significant changes in the legal and public policy arenas. It is also less vulnerable to being discounted if the value or belief is called into question by counterarguments, though as we shall see, this is still a problem for professional sexual exploitation (Ibarre and Kitsuse, 1993; Snow and Benford, 1988).

The process I describe here is an illustration of domain expansion or frame extension and amplification (Best, 1990; Snow et al., 1986). I argue that in the case of the framing of professional sexual exploitation, such an expansion is an attempt to render the frame more effective in the social problem marketplace and therefore strategically more useful. Best (1990) implies that expansion can make a claim more radical and therefore less effective (see also Jenness, 1995). Snow et al. (1986), by contrast, suggest that the process works on both an individual and organizational level and is used strategically to draw on frame resonance or augment frame potency. This chapter describes the various ways in which this expansion has taken place, using examples both from professional sexual misconduct itself and, for comparison, from other related areas.

Best's (1990) natural history approach has shown that domain expansion goes through several stages. The first involves the initial claims-making where an issue is framed self-consciously to convince the relevant audiences that there is, indeed, a social problem. In the second stage, the issue is accepted as a social problem by others and moves onto the policy agenda as a problem about which "something must be done." The final stage in Best's natural history sees the established claim expanded to include new, related claims under the umbrella of the original claim. Just as traditional rape (the stranger in a dark alley) has been expanded to include acquaintance rape, date rape, and marital rape, so, too, has professional sexual exploitation been expanded to take in a broader range of victims, professionals, and exploitative situations.

Best (1990) suggests that claims-makers have an interest in domain expansion (78). To the extent that claims compete for attention, recognition, funding, and other scarce resources, claims-makers have an interest in suggesting that what might otherwise be considered new claims are, in fact, examples of the original claim. Best points out, however, that domain expansion can have negative effects in the social problems marketplace because the credibility that attached to the narrower claim does not extend to its expanded form (82–86). In the case of professional sexual misconduct the effect has been the opposite; it has made the claim *more* credible to the audiences to whom it is addressed. It is thus more consistent with Snow et al.'s (1986: 472) description of frame alignment to "extend the boundaries of its (the movement's) primary framework so as to encompass interests and points of view that are incidental to its primary objectives but of considerable salience to potential adherents," though some might argue that whether the expansion is considered incidental depends on which adherents are involved.

THE FRAMES OF REFERENCE

When the phenomenon of professional sexual exploitation was most recently constructed about 20 years ago, it focused on sexual exploitation in therapeutic relationships and was a part of the women's movement of that period (e.g., Chesler, 1972). Under this construction, the paradigmatic case was that of a strong male professional exploiting a female patient or client who came to him in need of professional care. Professional sexual exploitation was located within the parameters of a number of claims of abuse of women. As one speaker at a conference phrased it: "There are many expressions of sexual politics. We began with stranger rape and moved to battery, date rape, acquaintance rape, women in pornography, sexual slavery; then children began with father/daughter child sexual abuse, grandfathers, extrafamilial abuse, victims younger and younger than we ever imagined" (Butler, 1994).

Another movement also gave impetus to the claim of professional sexual exploitation, that of the medical consumer movement (see Starr, 1982). In that frame the emphasis was on the inappropriate treatment of patients in a medical setting. Patients in therapy were more willing to question their therapists' behavior and less willing to accept at face value their explanations of that behavior (Bohmer, 1994).

As the claim expanded, however, it took in a broader range of professions, situations, and types of victim, some of whom were no longer represented by the frames from either the women's movement or the medical consumer movement. This is particularly true for those abused by the clergy, whose cases began to come to light in the 1980s and where the claim is part of a challenge to the unquestioned power of the church (see, e.g., Fortune, 1989; Berry, 1992; Jenkins, 1995). In addition, each of the frames (the feminist and the medical) has problems gaining acceptance by the various audiences to whom the frame is addressed.

The limitation of the medical frame is that it sidesteps professional sexual exploitation's natural place in the universe of female victimization, even though the vast majority of those who are exploited sexually as adults by professionals are women (Bouhoutsos et al., 1983; Gonsiorek et al., 1994). Also, the medical frame is less able to benefit from gains made in other claims that primarily affect women, like domestic violence and rape.

The limitation of a frame that comes out of the women's movement lies in the ambivalent social attitudes toward women and their behavior, especially in the current political climate. Claims-makers of professional sexual exploitation as a "woman's issue" are faced with an inherent contradiction. They can define the woman as a victim buffeted by forces beyond her control and at the mercy of the professional. If they do this, they are caught up in all the pejorative aspects of this dependent female role, in which the claim is dismissed as "just a woman's problem." To claim that a professional is sexually exploiting his patient, client, or parishioner seems to imply that she has no power or ability to decide for herself whether or not to engage in the sexual relationship.

Alternatively, one can define the woman as someone just like a man, that is, a person responsible for her behavior. If the claim is that a woman is not indecisive, dependent, and easily coerced but instead fully adult and responsible, then how can one say that she has been exploited? How can professional sexual exploitation be constructed to avoid the charge made in episodes of date rape that a consensual, sexual relationship is involved? This conflict is clearly shown in the legislative debates about criminalizing therapist–patient sex, in which many legislators continue to see the issue as one of consent. In Massachusetts even the local Civil Liberties Union has objected to the proposed legislation on the ground that a law that does not allow a woman to consent to sexual behavior in therapeutic situations is "demeaning to women" (Gardner, 1995).

THE COMBINED, EXPANDED FRAMEWORK

Recently, advocates have attempted to develop a more effective frame as a way of combining and expanding upon the two original frames of reference of professional sexual exploitation. This frame expands the domain of each of the others in a way that minimizes the limitations and strategic problems of the earlier frames. It leads to a more effective frame that can be linked to several widely held beliefs (Snow and Benford, 1988). This is particularly important in a case such as this that relies on acceptance by a variety of established institutions as well as members of interest groups. The potential result of such an expansion contrasts with the domain expansion described by Best (1990) in which new, peripheral (and probably more radical) claims are piggybacked onto the original problem with the risk that the previous consensus about the problem will collapse. The expanded frame that I call the medical/professional/power framework does not, on the whole, deal directly with the issue of gender. Instead, it links the claim to the abuse of power with the gender-connected cultural meanings of power imbalances inherent in relationships such as those under discussion. I do not claim that this makes the claim itself "nongendered." The legal system, one of the major audiences for claims of professional sexual exploitation, does, however, behave as if there is a "nongendered" way of framing this claim despite the development of a feminist jurisprudence arguing otherwise. Constitutional developments in the last two decades have, for the most part, stressed the importance of "gender-neutrality" in the law, ignoring gender differences (see Lindgren and Taub, 1994: 106–43). Thus, a frame that does not deal directly with gender can be more effective in the legal arena.

Expanding the frame as a medical/professional/power issue has several strategic benefits as well as some risks. It serves the traditional claims-making goals of making the problem look bigger and therefore more serious (see Best, 1990). It takes in more victims, professionals, and situations. It also offers a ready-made set of remedies. As long as the relevant professions accept the construction of professional sexual misconduct as a "problem," it can be added as domain expansion to the list of all kinds of unprofessional and unethical behavior and treated accordingly. Professional organizations and the legal system already have in place mechanisms for the processing of complaints of unprofessional or unethical behavior. The expanded frame addresses the issue of gender by bringing in power as its stand-in. It thus seeks to avoid the negative aspects of a claim, which can be dismissed as "only a woman's problem," while, nevertheless, emphasizing the ways in which women are especially vulnerable to the behavior. It links the frame to several widely held beliefs, including the medical exhortation *primum non nocere*, the belief that appropriate services should be provided in return for the payment of a fee and that one should not take advantage of the needy. It also draws in clergy abuse, which may not otherwise fit into either the women's movement or the medical consumer model. For example, one scholar places the recent publicity about clergy abuse within the framework of an increase in anti-Catholic public attitudes (Jenkins, 1995, 1996). The frame expansion at work here thus makes the claim more salient and potentially less radical, rather than the reverse. The risk is that it will not be perceived as one claim but, rather, that each of the elements will be perceived as a separate and therefore less significant claim. As later chapters show, there is some evidence that this has happened, which may have contributed to the movement's lack of success as a social change agent.

Following are the specific ways in which the frame of reference is expanded.

Extending the Range of Potential Victims

Claims-makers expand the frame by asserting that anyone can be the subject of professional sexual misconduct, not just dependent, weak women (Luepker and Retsch-Bogart, 1986; Vinson, 1984; Holstein and

Miller, 1990). Potential victims thus include not only all women but also men (Bouhoutsos et al., 1983). Extending the focus to sexual exploitation other than the traditional male professional–female victim variety does, however, mask the important fact mentioned earlier that, like rape and domestic violence, in the case of adults, this is primarily a problem of men harming women. Professional sexual exploitation of adult males and same-sex exploitation do, indeed, exist, though these forms of the behavior are much rarer (Bouhoutsos et al., 1983). Experts maintain that, recently, more men have complained of being exploited, though it is hard to know whether this indicates a change in the pattern of professional sexual exploitation or part of the increased willingness to make such claims public (It's Never O.K., 1994). Those who treat victims of professional sexual misconduct believe, however, that men are sexually exploited at a higher rate than incidence statistics would suggest, though still at a rate far lower than for women (Gonsiorek et al., 1994). The case of Dr. Margaret Bean-Bayog, accused of a sexual relationship with her male patient, received extensive publicity and may have been taken as an indication that sexual exploitation by a female professional toward a male victim happens frequently, though, in fact, it is the least frequent combination (Gonsiorek et al., 1994; "Psychotherapy," 1992; Butterfield, 1992b; McNamara, 1994). Some argue that the media are more interested in male victims, on the assumption that men must suffer more, as well as a belief that things that happen to men are simply more interesting (Cole, 1994). The interest may, in fact, be because female-to-male professional sexual exploitation reverses traditional power/gender relationships. Similarly, the media are interested in the (statistically) rare cases of battered males and the sexual harassment of males (e.g., Crichton, 1994). The "distortion" from the publicity surrounding celebrated, though infrequent, cases may have helped efforts of those wishing to cast claims in "nongendered" terms.

The potential victim pool is also extended by including people of both sexes who are indirectly involved in professional sexual exploitation. This includes spouses and children and even wives of perpetrators (described as the silent victims at one conference) among those harmed (Luepker, 1995; Milgrom, 1989b). As a result, support groups have been set up to cater to the needs of these associate victims (Luepker and O'Brien, 1989). One newsletter for victims expressly included what are called pro-survivors, defined as "supportive relatives, friends or significant others of survivors" (*Survivor Activist* 2.4 [1994]). In the case of clergy sexual abuse, the congregation has been included in the definition of victims (Maris and McDonough, 1995). Some claims-makers even expand the frame to cover everyone who deals with the issue, though that is unusual. One person at the It's Never O.K. conference said that "we are all survivors, of the patriarchal system."

Frame expansion for the purpose of membership in self-help groups includes as a victim anyone who considers herself to have been exploited

(Bohmer, 1995a). Self-defined victims included those who were raped, those for whom the sexual relationship did not include intercourse or took place after therapy ended, one whose claim was 30 years old, one who married her "perpetrator" and lived with him for a number of years, and those who were not abused sexually but whose claim is based on emotional abuse. All these people consider their claims valid, and many of them are actively involved in making them public.

The expanded medical/professional/power framework has benefited from the extensive recent publicity about sexual abuse by members of the clergy, which has primarily involved male children rather than adult males. As one professional in the field told me: "It's a good add-on because kids and male victims are involved" (Schoener, 24 June 1993). From the point of view of the claims-makers, this "add-on" helps make it clear to the public that professional sexual exploitation is not "just" a problem involving male perpetrators and female victims or one involving only therapists and their patients. This is particularly helpful, as the claims against the Catholic Church for child sexual abuse have been more successful in the public arena than other parts of the frame (Jenkins, 1995).

Extending the Pool of Abusers

The original claim of therapist–patient sexual exploitation has been expanded to include a variety of other professionals from lawyers to massage therapists. Some claims-makers expand the domain even further by arguing that anyone can be an abuser. At one conference the phrase "we are all abusers" became something of a leitmotif for the meeting (Restoring the Integrity, 1993). Included were not only those who actually exploit patients and clients but also those who "abuse" patients by ignoring their claims of having been abused or do not take the claims sufficiently seriously, or use the claims for their own ends (like some lawyers and therapists) or even by being part of a system in which such exploitation is possible.

The Abuse of Power

Power is connected to the claims-making process in professional sexual exploitation in various ways. In addition to the power imbalance inherent in male–female interactions and adult–child interactions, there is the power imbalance inherent in the professional relationship. The expanded medical/professional/power frame of reference diminishes the focus on sexuality and the male–female power imbalance by stressing power imbalance in its various forms. This has its parallel in the construction of other problems that primarily harm women. Rape is constructed as power and violence rather than sex, and sexual harassment is likewise connected to the power imbalance in academe and the workplace.

This abuse of power theme is evident from the statement of one victim who said: "I am a survivor of sexual exploitation by a therapist. I want to share with you some of the vivid sexual aspects of the relationship with my therapist. But this is not about sex, it is about power. Keep that in mind, because sex is only a tool in all this" (Wohlberg, 1993). Or, as another victim put it: "It's not about sex, but power. I mean, have you ever met him? So it's power—that the rules don't apply to him" (Lehr, 1994: 1).

Another victim provided a graphic description of the nature of the power her clergyman had over her. "He asked me to destroy the pictures (of another female parishioner wearing only seductive lingerie). I did it, I did anything. I'd have drunk Kool-Aid if he'd asked me. I was already trapped by his spell" (Carol, 1993). Those who are exploited by the clergy are, in general, anxious to stress that the issue is about power and not about religion, perhaps in the hope of not destroying religious beliefs in the victims.

In one case, the nature of the exploitation itself indicated that the victim's experience had, as she stated, "very little to do with sex" (Park, 1994). When she testified during the malpractice trial, she described the details of the oral sex she performed on her therapist. She was asked whether her therapist was sitting or standing, and when she said that he was standing, the expert witness pointed out that the therapist was therefore "on a power trip." The victim said in an interview: "Sex was the vehicle. With someone else, he may have pushed his power in a different way, but because I was a sitting duck, an incest survivor, that was the logical way to proceed with me" (Park, 1994).

That the power being abused is professional is made clear in one victim's statement about what happened to her as a teenager in therapy. "I had absolutely no knowledge of what was proper or improper in therapy. My parents didn't know anything or provide guidance. He was able to use the role of being an expert over me" (Sharon, 1993).

Another case illustrates that the abuse of professional power can be intentional on the part of the abuser. A podiatrist who was being sued for abusing a teenage girl appeared in court wearing his white coat, the classic symbol of medical power and expertise (Roseman, 1997).

One public official used abuse of power rhetoric by connecting it with the rhetoric of entitlement (Ibarre and Kitsuse, 1993). She linked professional sexual exploitation to the right to health care, a central part of the consumer health movement. She said: "Sexual exploitation is an abuse of power that shatters the trusting relationship that there needs to be if healing is to occur. . . . Health care is a right. Abuse of the patient or client is abuse of the health care system" (Grier, 1994).

One of the ways in which the abuse of power theme can be used involves the quintessential patriarchal analogy, that of incest. Since patients experience the therapeutic relationship as symbolic of the relationship

with their parents, a sexual relationship with the patient is seen as a violation akin to incest (Benowitz, 1991). As one woman described her situation
with her therapist: "He was Daddy. That's why I didn't want to have sex
with him. He was my father. You don't have sex with your father"
(D'Addario, 1977: 346). Another woman described the experience as
"making love to my father" (*Task Force*, 1991). A bumper sticker in the
parking lot at the 1997 Linkup conference said "Clergy Sex Abuse Is
Incest." For Pagano, sexual exploitation by a therapist is also financial exploitation. She describes it as "incest with a professional twist, incorporat-
ing all the debilitating dynamics of the familial variety but for a fee"
(1997a: 23).

Characterizing the exploitation as incest connects the power rhetoric
back to gender indirectly because incest is so often a father–daughter problem. At the same time it provides a basis for including in the frame sexual
abuse of children by members of the clergy, which in many cases arises out
of surrogate parental relationships.

The abuse of power framework is closely linked to the role of transference in the therapeutic relationship that affects patients of either sex
(Greenson, 1967). Because of the nature of transference, a patient in therapy is not in a position to consent to a sexual relationship with her therapist as she would in any other adult relationship. A therapist who engages
in a sexual relationship with a patient is therefore abusing the power
he has as a result of the transference. This claim is much easier to make
with reference to those involved in a therapeutic relationship than it is
for other forms of professional relationships like lawyer–client or pastor–parishioner. Those framing the problem with respect to these latter
professions have attempted to resolve this issue by maintaining that a
pseudotransference situation also exists in these relationships. They argue
that, for example, at least some clients of lawyers are very much like patients, who are not equal to the professional in status and power but who
become dependent and may have feelings very similar to the feelings
caused by the transference process that characterizes therapist–patient relationships (Firestone and Simon, 1992: 682–85).

This argument is clearly more successful with certain types of clients
than with others. A female divorce client, for example, is the classic case
of a client who seeks help at a particularly vulnerable time in her life. For
many women, their relationship with their divorce lawyer has many of the
characteristics of a therapist–patient relationship. Just as in a therapeutic
situation, a female divorce client reveals personal secrets and relies heavily on her lawyer's advice and assistance. The professional who takes advantage of this vulnerability and reliance is thereby abusing his power
over his client.

For some, an expanded medical/professional/power framework makes
possible domain expansion beyond that of sexual exploitation to all kinds

of emotional exploitation in professional relationships. It includes other behavior, such as verbal sexual behavior, having a patient work for the professional, or, as in one case of a lawyer–client relationship, having a client pose for nude photographs. It can even extend to the "tone" of the relationship in which the victim defines it as emotional abuse without any specific behavioral indicators.

The abuse of power theme in emotional abuse can also be connected to force, a spillover from the social construction of rape. One therapist used the term "mind rape" to describe nonsexual abuse in therapy, thereby linking the power issue back to the power inherent in forcible rape (Brown, 1994a). Like the social construction of rape itself, the description she gives of the circumstances in which "mind rape" occurs does not stress the sexual aspects of the behavior. Instead, the focus is on more general power-related issues: "It happens when the therapist is dishonest, when they fail to tell what they know, when the therapist doesn't have a clear frame, when they break the frame whatever it is, when the person is objectified" (Brown, 1994a). When asked if she saw it as a gender issue or a power issue, Brown (1994b) said that she saw it as "a power issue, not a gender issue. Both male and female therapists have done it."

The parallel use of the term "rape" in the context of clergy sexual misconduct is that of "spiritual rape," used by a victim at the 1997 Linkup conference. Here, instead of connecting the rape to therapeutic exploitation of the mind, it is connected to the exploitation of religious belief. Other victims connect their abuse with other negative experiences; one called it soul murder, thereby connecting it to another violent crime. Another called it emotional adultery, which captures the sense of illicitness, though not the violence or emotional abuse.

The expansion of the frame of professional sexual abuse to include emotional abuse illustrates problems inherent in attempting to deal with diverse audiences in its construction. This type of domain expansion is more analogous to the traditional pattern in which the addition of a more radical claim can have the effect of breaking down the consensus about the nature of the problem, especially among some of the audiences for the frame. For example, one victim who was involved in what she called "a very sexualized" therapeutic relationship without actual sexual contact spoke of the difficulties of finding a lawyer to file civil suits in cases such as hers. "It's hard to find a lawyer, because they are not interested if it isn't sexual. . . . They say juries don't understand emotional abuse" (Phyllis, 1993).

Boundary Violations

A further way the claim can be expanded is by focusing on the responsibility of the professional to avoid violating boundaries in the therapist–patient relationship. In this context, sexual exploitation is part of a more general claim of boundary violation. This argument is much easier to make in the therapeutic situation, where there is a body of scholarship that points out the dangers of boundary violations in general (Peterson, 1992). Thus, it is unethical, as well as bad therapy, for example, to use a patient to do typing or baby-sitting or to socialize with her outside the therapy. Those who work in the field point out that in most cases where there is a sexual relationship, other kinds of boundary violations also exist, thereby making this a practical as well as theoretical option for construction of the claim (Jorgenson, Bishing, and Sutherland, 1992). One victim in telling her story described a series of connections she had with two therapists, including living with one of them: "[T]here was no sexual involvement but she had made it clear that she and her husband would be interested." The victim's second therapist told her about the illness of his wife, cried in the therapy sessions, had her buy books for him, kissed and hugged her, and used as his own lawyer one of the members of the group in which the victim also participated. "I was not interested in him as a lover. . . . he looked like a fat Norman Schwarzkopf." Instead, she viewed the behavior as boundary violations, all of which featured in her civil lawsuit against the therapist (Laverne, 1993).

The boundary violation framework has a special benefit for those representing plaintiffs in civil lawsuits against professionals because it avoids the problem which arises when insurance companies refuse to cover malpractice claims against therapists who engage in sexual relationships. Therapists are usually insured for "professional services rendered," and insurance companies argue that sexual conduct is not part of the professional services, though a number of courts have disagreed with this view (Jorgenson, Bishing, and Sutherland, 1992). In addition, some insurance carriers have exclusions in their policies that explicitly deny recovery for sexual behavior. Lawyers for victims of professional sexual exploitation may, therefore, need to argue that the malpractice stemmed from acts other than the sexual conduct itself. Boundary violations serve this purpose for the legal audience for the claim.

The rhetoric of boundary violation has also been used in a broader context. One speaker at the It's Never O.K. conference used the term "breaking and entering" as an idiom for professional sexual exploitation. Here the behavior is analogized to a property boundary violation (Butler, 1994). This is an effective domain expansion, as it plugs into our fears of having the boundaries of our property violated and uses the symbols of the criminal law to imply an appropriate remedy. The ultimate "boundary violation" analogy was used by one activist who called the sexual abuse of children by priests "murder of youngsters' minds" (Fitzpatrick, 1996).

The use of the boundary violation framework in constructing professional sexual exploitation is not without its critics, however. The need for boundaries is one of the major tenets of traditional psychotherapy (Peterson, 1992). Recently, however, this formulation has been criticized because of its connection to the hierarchy of traditional (male) power (Heywood, 1993). Heywood (1994) argues that boundaries "provide the protection of patriarchally structured power relationships" and describes her experience in therapy as one in which "the therapist used the concept of boundaries to distance me." Heywood (1994) calls it "rigid boundary fundamentalism." Boundary violations are here linked to traditionalism and gender and discredited.

Betrayal/Breach of Trust

Closely related to the abuse of power and the boundary violation framework is the claim that sexual contact between a professional and a client can stem from, and result in, an abuse or breach of trust. For example, the television movie of Barbara Noel's book about sexual abuse by her psychiatrist was called *Betrayal of Trust*, and the book by Julie Roy of her experience at the hands of her psychiatrist was called *Betrayal* (Noel with Watterson, 1992; Freeman and Roy, 1976). An important recent scholarly book on the subject is called *Breach of Trust* (Gonsiorek, 1994), while another is called *Betrayal of Trust* (Friedman and Boumil, 1995). This focus is especially powerful in the case of lawyer–client sexual contact. The logic is that a sexual relationship may involve an unfair exploitation of the lawyer's fiduciary position and may impair the lawyer's ability to represent the client. A fiduciary relationship is said to exist "when one person justifiably places confidence in another whose aid, advice, or protection is sought in some matter" (Jorgenson, 1995b: 239). The focus is, in part, on the financial damage that a client may suffer by becoming involved sexually with the person who is also acting in the capacity of her financial adviser. For example, a divorce client who is involved in an unwanted sexual relationship with her lawyer is more likely to accept a quick settlement of her claim rather than to wait for one that is financially more advantageous to her. In one case in which an attorney was disciplined for his sexual behavior with a client, the court said: "The attorney stands in a fiduciary relationship with the client. . . . By making unsolicited sexual advances to a client, an attorney perverts the very essence of the lawyer–client relationship" (*In re Gibson*, 1985: 699–700). In another case, the judge said a sexual relationship between attorney and client "can undermine the lawyer's professional integrity and judgment and dishonor the client's trust" ("People v. Boyer," 1997). Breach of a fiduciary relationship in a sexual context locks in directly with other breaches of fiduciary duty. Thus, it provides credibility to the expanded medical/professional/power framework by linking it to other unprofessional behavior by lawyers.

Moral Failings

Some who focus on sexual exploitation among the clergy define the behavior in moral or spiritual terms (e.g., Fortune, 1989). A pastor who has
engaged in sexual behavior with a parishioner is seen to have fallen from
the moral standards set for him by the church. One lawyer who works on
cases of clergy sexual exploitation pointed out that this used to be an even
more common construction than it is now, where the behavior was a moral
failing that could be corrected by prayer (Shiltz, 1993). This focus puts the
claim in a category with other moral lapses of the clergy, like alcohol or
drug use or financial misconduct, and also serves to remove it from considerations of gender.

COUNTERCLAIMS AND BACKLASH

Counterclaims that deny the validity of allegations of claims-makers
have surfaced in the process of constructing professional sexual exploitation. For the most part, these counterclaims fit into Ibarre and Kitsuse's
(1993) category of unsympathetic counterrhetoric, as they deny both the
characterization of the claim and accordingly the remedies. There are three
different types of unsympathetic counterrhetoric used in this context.
First, there is the counterclaim that does not dispute the existence of the
events on which the claim is based, but rather its characterization as a social problem. For example, one counterclaim paints the women who claim
to have been sexually exploited as consenting adults who "had an affair"
that turned sour, instead of as victims of sexual exploitation. In this counterargument, the relationship must have been consensual; otherwise, the
victim would have walked away from the professional relationship.
Similarly, those constructing domestic violence as a social problem are
asked why a battered woman did not leave the battering relationship.
Those who wish to expand the domain of rape to include date rape confront the counterrhetoric that the victim should not have gone to the apart-
ment or out on the date and that the allegations of rape are simply
morning-after regrets or misunderstandings (Roiphe, 1993; Collison,
1992). The issue of why a woman who complains of sexual harassment did
not simply turn down the offer of a sexual relationship is a central element
of those counterclaims. In all these cases, the counterrhetoric places the behavior in the category of ordinary (and acceptable) sexual interaction
rather than abuse. This divergence of construction is made clear in the
phrase used by one respondent, referring to a leader in the field of clergy
sexual abuse: "In Marie Fortune's world, there's no such thing as a consensual affair" (Shiltz, 1993). This counterclaim may prove effective because many of the victims themselves, at least initially, define the
encounter as a consensual one (Bohmer, 1994). One woman reported that

it was not until eight years after the relationship took place that her definition of what happened changed. "At the time I thought of it as an affair"
(Terry, 1993). In addition, some victims find themselves in love with the
professional. As one victim put it: "I called it a relationship. I felt I was in
love with him" (*Crossing the Boundaries*, 1992: 11). Evelyn Walker says of
her relationship with her therapist: "I felt he truly loved me. He would always be there; he told me he would be" (Walker and Young, 1986: 72).
Claims-makers argue that these perceptions do not indicate genuine consent, the linchpin of the counterrhetoric. Rather, they are a result of the
professional's manipulation of the transference reinforced by his statements and his behavior.

A variant of this counterclaim comes from those who recognize the past
validity of the claim but who assert that the problem no longer exists. This
is a strategy of the church, which in the face of the overwhelming evidence
about child sexual abuse by priests belatedly admitted that there was a
problem. Now, however, they frame the problem as that of a "few bad apples" who have been appropriately dealt with by the church authorities
(Anderson, 1996).

The second type of counterclaim accepts the narrowest variant of the
claim, while denying the validity of the expanded version. While the public may be willing to accept the "worst" examples of professional sexual
exploitation, the expansion of the claim may result in counterrhetoric.
Those who are actually raped in therapy or placed under the influence of
drugs and then exploited are much more acceptable as victims than those
who have what may look like a consensual sexual relationship with a
lawyer or with their therapist after the therapy has ended (however much
they might have been coerced by the therapist). Children are the quintes-
sentially innocent victims who by definition (legal and literal) cannot consent to sex, so their claims are seen as "real." This may, in part, account for
the greater apparent acceptance of clergy sexual misconduct, though even
here, juries have difficulty imagining the plaintiff as a child in cases that
are not tried until the victim is an adult (Roseman, 1997).

The case of rape provides a useful analogy. It has been expanded from
the classic "stranger in a dark alley" situation to other events, like date
rape and the rape of women who have a "reputation" for sexual promiscuity. Date rape has generated the latest wave of publicity, asserting that
women cry rape when in fact they have regrets about consensual sex the
morning after (e.g., Roiphe, 1993). In the same way, quid pro quo sexual
harassment in which a woman loses her job because she is unwilling to
meet the sexual demands of her boss is much more acceptable than hostile environment sexual harassment in which a woman claims that her life
as an employee was made impossible by the environment in which she
had to work. While this latter form clearly falls within the legal definition
of sexual harassment (*Harris* v. *Forklift Systems, Inc.*, 1993), this is the

harassment that many men "just don't get" (Riger, 1991). This counter-rhetoric is concordant with the traditional view of women, in which those whose behavior defines them as "real" victims are accepted as victims, while those whose behavior challenges what is considered acceptable female behavior are not.

A similar strategy is used by the church in its response to claims of child sexual abuse. It has redefined the category as one that includes only adolescents, rather than children, which bolsters the counterclaim mentioned before that the problem has been dealt with (Economous, 1996). They claim that church-run treatment facilities have had tremendous success in treating the few wayward priests, though no research has been permitted by outside scholars (Isely, 1996).

The third strategy, however, goes further by denying the very existence of professional sexual exploitation and asserting, instead, that the claim itself is a fabrication. Charges are supposedly made up as a way of getting back at the professional for some reason or another. For example, it is argued that the victim is not happy with the outcome of the professional relationship (she lost her lawsuit, the marriage for which she was being counseled failed anyway, or the professional terminated the relationship when she wanted it to continue). This has its parallel in rape cases in which the woman is seen in terms Rosemarie Tong (1984: 100–102) calls the "lying temptress," who contrives false charges out of some psychological disorder or for personal revenge. In both cases, this counterrhetoric turns the powerful person in the encounter, the alleged rapist or professional, into the victim, a role that often generates great sympathy for him and little for the alleged victim.

A variant of this "fabrication" claim comes about when a person in therapy reclaims memories of a long-repressed abusive sexual relationship. As extensive recent publicity indicates, the alternative view is that these memories themselves are fabrications generated by the efforts of overly enthusiastic therapists, in what has become known as the "false memory syndrome" (Crews, 1994). While claims of false memory syndrome have usually arisen in incest cases, there have also been cases in which the claims have been of professional sexual exploitation (primarily by members of the clergy), as the following examples illustrate.

A case brought against a bishop by two women in Minnesota was dropped when it became clear that the allegations were false. The attorney for the bishop argued that the women's therapist was responsible for "planting false memories" (Allen, 1993). The filing of a $10 million lawsuit against Cardinal Joseph Bernardin in November 1993, which was later withdrawn, also illustrates the difficulties posed by "repressed memories" in constructing this social problem. Steven Cook, the plaintiff, had apparently "recovered" memories of the alleged sexual abuse by Cardinal

Bernardin under hypnosis by "an unlicensed therapist trained on weekends at a school founded by a New Age guru" (Lewis, 1994).

The significance of the false memory syndrome for the claims-making process lies in the extent of its generalizability. Those constructing professional sexual exploitation as a social problem usually recognize the existence of mistaken claims but argue that a few false cases disprove neither the existence of the problem nor the ability of a person to recover repressed memories in therapy (Herman and Harvey, 1993). Some proponents of false memory syndrome argue, however, that the existence of the syndrome indicates that the social problem as constructed by claims-makers does not exist. The Bernardin case, because of its widespread publicity, gives support to this view, as people may assume that this case is just one example of a widespread phenomenon. Combined with other, well-publicized cases of successful suits against therapists, it has been effective in bolstering the position of the church in its counterclaims that the problem is really not very serious (Anderson, 1996).

Connected to the false memory syndrome is a general view that people (especially women) who are in therapy are crazy and that their allegations must be dismissed as the psychotic ravings of the disturbed. It took one woman seven years before she could get the Florida Board of Medicine to take action against a prominent Miami psychiatrist who had sexually exploited her, "Throughout history, those of us who report sexual abuse have been treated as psychotic, labeled hysteric, portrayed as promiscuous and dismissed as expendable" (Gentry, 1993).

While the counterrhetoric is not always stated in specific gender terms, the implication is that it is most likely women, because of their particular "nature" (i.e., hysterical, conniving) who make such false claims. The Bernardin case does provide some counterweight to this by illustrating that it is not only women who are alleged to fabricate claims.

The counterrhetoric also attempts to redefine the motivation of the claims-makers themselves in pejorative terms. They are labeled "sex-hating feminists" who are out to victimize men by their claims of professional sexual exploitation, thereby challenging the traditional patriarchal order. Sometimes this redefinition is accomplished by discrediting the claims-maker in some fashion. The woman who subsequently treated Melissa Roberts, whose case of professional sexual exploitation was the subject of a *Frontline* program, herself suffered significant harassment by the lawyers for the defendant ("My Doctor, My Lover," 1993). Her practice suffered as a result of the negative publicity she received to the point where she decided to move out of the area. The jury in this case found the defendant responsible for the sexual exploitation, but in his interview on *Frontline*, he asserted that he had suffered no reduction in the number of referrals from his colleagues, nor was his reputation harmed.

As we have seen, most of the counterarguments are in response to the framing of the issue as a "woman's" issue, which fits with Jenkins' assertion that the framing of clergy sexual abuse has been a success (1995, 1996). One of the benefits of the expanded frame described earlier is that it deflects attention from the "woman's" aspect of the issue and provides arguments to counter the counterarguments. For example, the counterargument that the sexual behavior is consensual can be answered by arguing that even so-called consensual sex has no place in professional relationships, especially among those of either gender who are in need of the help offered by the professional. This response to the counterrhetoric asserts that claimants are not "sex-hating feminists" or out to discredit the church but people concerned about boundaries and abuse of power in all professional relationships. People who were abused by professionals, especially as children, have repressed their memories because they were too intolerable to retain. The repressed memories cannot be dismissed as the fabrications of crazy people but a natural response to the seriousness of the issue. All these arguments to counter the counterarguments are made easier by the broader range of victims, professionals, and situations covered by the expanded frame.

CONCLUSION

Claims-makers arguing that professional sexual exploitation is a social problem have made efforts to bring the issue to public attention and to generate some activity in the political and legal arena designed to do something about it. As we see in later chapters, they have not been very successful. Even the clergy abuse claim has had more success as a claim than as a social movement resulting in significant social change. There remain tensions among claims-makers for "ownership" of this problem (Best, 1990). As we have seen, some claims-makers frame it as one example of the series of issues where women are the primary victims, while others frame it as a violation of the doctor–patient relationship, and still others as a religious issue. This lack of consensus appears to have contributed to the lack of success of the narrow frames. Combining them into the expanded medical/professional/power frame offers social movement strategists the hope that an effective frame will be accepted by the public as well as the legal and regulatory audiences on whom the claims-makers depend for recognition and remedies. They may be able to move this from the category of "other people's business" to one that is seen as a threat to all of us who rely on professional help in a wide variety of contexts. The expanded frame has a wider potential audience and is linked to several core values held by that audience. Accordingly, it has greater mobilizing potential and is more likely to hold up in the face of the counterarguments that have been raised. It attempts to encompass the widest range of diverse values and to avoid the perception that it is too narrow to resonate with a wide audience.

While the expanded claim can avoid the still-prevalent conflicting attitudes to problems where women are the primary victims, it does women a disservice by reinforcing traditional views of women rather than pushing for changes in social attitudes. Framing it as a "women's issue" has the benefit of spillover from gains made by the women's movement in drawing attention to the victimization of women.

Such an approach also risks being perceived not as one broad, important social problem but rather as several, each with different goals and potential remedies. As we shall see, there is some evidence that clergy sexual abuse and therapist sexual abuse are still considered separate and distinct social problems. This is one of the factors that, it may be argued, have contributed to the relative lack of success activists have had using the frame as the basis of a social movement.

NOTE

1. The different terminology is characteristic of this field, which has been developed both by social problem theorists and social movement theorists, with relatively little overlap between the two fields. The terminology used in this chapter reflects both fields.

—3—

THE VICTIMS

I called it a relationship. I felt I was in love with him. I now understand the power imbalance and how destructive it was for me.
—*Crossing the Boundaries*, 1992

Gradually, I have developed real anger and outrage at what happened. I finally realized I had had no opportunity to say no to his sexual invitation. . . . I had no other choice. When I felt angry I could see myself as a victim rather than a stupid participant.
—Rutter, 1989

INTRODUCTION

Just as professional sexual exploitation must be recognized as a social and legal problem to become part of the public agenda, so, too, must the individual come to believe that she has been wronged. This chapter shows how the issue is framed on an individual level, using the literature of the transformation of disputes (Felstiner et al., 1981) and that of cognitive schemata (e.g., Fiske and Taylor, 1983). Felstiner et al. argue that for a dispute to become a legal claim it must go through a transformation process of "naming, blaming, and claiming" in which an individual comes to recognize that she has been victimized and then takes steps to do something about it. I identify these stages in this process and some of the triggers for these stages.

The first stage of this transformation process is the definition by the injured party of her status as victim. The definition of a victim varies depending on who is doing the defining and why. It also has important implications for the changes that take place as a victim goes through the process. Social psychologists argue that the cognitive schemata that the individual and society apply to the definition of the events giving rise to the status of victim are also significant. These are the assumptions we all hold about other people that enable us to function (Fiske and Taylor, 1983: 139). Our choice of social schemata affects the way we process new information (Fiske and Taylor, 1983). The schema chosen also affects which "scripts" we choose for acting on the information. Thus, a victim will engage in certain behavior depending on which cognitive schema she applies to the events in question. This chapter shows why and how different people select different schemata to characterize the scripts for action in the process of transforming an event into a legally actionable injury.

There are several forms of overt action a victim can take once she has defined the event as one of victimization. They are not mutually exclusive. They range from a criminal claim to a civil lawsuit to several forms of administrative action, including filing a complaint to the ethics board of a professional organization or a licensing board, or, an informal confrontation with her perpetrator. The fact that all of the formal options are almost invariably long and complex is, as we shall see, an essential element of the pattern of choices made by the victim throughout the process.

THE VICTIMS

Many victims of all kinds of sexual abuse do not report their abuse (FBI, 1982: 14). Why that is so has been the subject of research and comment (Koss and Harvey, 1991; Holmstrom and Burgess, 1983: 55–60). While it is even more difficult to obtain statistical data in the case of professional sexual misconduct, it seems likely that an even smaller proportion of women report their exploitation than report other forms of sexual abuse. In one study, researchers found that 96 percent of cases of patient–therapist involvement were not reported (Bouhoutsos et al., 1983). Of the 208 people who called a toll-free hot line set up by the College of Physicians and Surgeons of British Columbia to investigate sexual misconduct by physicians, only 23 had reported the incident to the college (*Crossing the Boundaries*, 1992: 65). The American Psychological Association reported 487 complaint inquiries for its membership of 73,263, resulting in 25 newly opened cases ("Report of the Ethics Committee," 1994).

Many victims never come to the recognition that they have been mistreated; many of them feel that they have been mistreated but have no idea that what took place was an ethical violation, let alone malpractice or (in some states) a criminal offense (Rutter, 1989). In one study, 80 percent of patients sexually abused by therapists did not know that they could initiate a civil or criminal action or that they could file a complaint with the state licensing board (Vinson, 1984). Even among those who know that there are avenues of redress available to them, they have at least as many reasons for not reporting as do their counterparts who have been raped

(*Crossing the Boundaries*, 1992; Pogrebin et al., 1992; Benowitz, 1991). Thus, for the majority of the victims of professional sexual misconduct, the script they choose is passive acceptance or personal recovery, rather than action.

The focus of this chapter is not, however, on those who do not report, for whatever reason, but rather on those few who do decide to respond. How do the victims who take action deal with the status of victim? How do they decide to define their situation in terms of the script for claimant? What process do they go through to become claimants rather than victims? What is the role of third parties in the process? Is the decision to take action connected to personal characteristics of the victim or events in the wider society? How are success and failure perceived by the victims themselves and by those in the social movement?

MEANING AND IMPLICATIONS OF THE VICTIM STATUS

The victimology literature, in general, assumes the definition of the term "victim," among other things, as one upon whom an act defined as criminal is perpetrated (Elias, 1986; Karmen, 1990). By contrast, feminists have cast aside the term "victim" as too dependent and now prefer the term "survivor" to describe a woman who has been raped or otherwise abused. As one author of a manual for victim assistance writes, "Activists in the social movement to stop victimization have begun to regard the term *victim* as pejorative, connoting relative weakness and powerlessness" (Andrews, 1992: 3). It is important to distinguish between the use of the word "victim" and the acceptance of the status implicit in the term.[1] Like so many other terms, this one has taken on a number of connotations not originally included in its meaning (Karmen, 1990). Because of the negative implications of the victim status, some of those who have been injured refuse to define themselves as victims.

As we shall see, this self-definition has behavioral implications in determining how someone responds. It does not, however, exist in a vacuum. It is linked to the beliefs and attributes that are related to the schemata of the role of victim of professional sexual exploitation (Fiske and Taylor, 1983). Thus, in choosing a script for action, the "victim" is influenced by the way others view the events that have taken place. By rejecting the definition of victim altogether, someone who has undergone a victimizing experience rejects those scripts that provide for efforts to claim redress. Before a victim becomes a claimant pursuing her claim, therefore, there must be both a self-definition and some agreement with this assessment by the wider society. There must also be some mechanism (most likely legal or administrative) within which the victim can make her claim.

For the victim of professional sexual misconduct, like the victim of any type of sexual abuse, the beliefs and attributes surrounding the events are both positive and negative. Thus, the victim can define herself and be defined by society as both a fool who brought the exploitation on herself and someone who has been grievously wronged by an abuse of power. Which of these schemata is more powerful determines whether she chooses the script of being passively acceptant or a claimant.

For victims whose injury is not based on sexual abuse, by contrast, the beliefs and attributes of the role may be positive and without the stigmatizing qualities mentioned before (e.g., Andrews, 1992; Gunn and Minch, 1988). For these victims, there is no need to replace the term or to deal with the conflicting implications of the status. For example, Durkin's research on victims of asbestos-related disease defines the status in positive, rather than stigmatizing, terms (Durkin, 1991).

Those victims of professional sexual exploitation who accept the passive and negative definition of "victim" may be anxious to throw it off as quickly as possible, for example, by replacing it with that of "survivor," which implies personal recovery. This emphasis is a central tenet of the social movement for professional sexual misconduct, which has the effect of limiting individual as well as social action. Those who define themselves as victims entitled to redress can move on from the definition of victim to that of claimant. In both cases the status of victim is a transitional one, accepted only until replaced by a different self-definition.

THE TRANSFORMATION PROCESS

Events That Give Rise to Victim Status: Naming

For a woman who has been involved in sexual misconduct by a professional, the acceptance of the status of victim represents the first stage in the process at which she can begin to see herself as a person with a grievance who is entitled to redress. It may not be necessary to use the word "victim" itself, with its positive and negative connotations, but some recognition of having been wronged is essential to the transformation process as well as the choice of an activist script for action.

For some women, the initial self-definition is as a participant who was responsible for what happened. "I kept blaming myself for having gotten myself into this situation, and after the experience with Rick, I felt awful about myself," one victim reported (Bass, 1989). Another said: "Gradually, I have developed real anger and outrage at what happened. I finally realized I had had no opportunity to say no to his sexual invitation. . . . I had had no other choice. When I felt angry I could see myself as a victim rather than a stupid participant" (Rutter, 1989: 123).

Some women never get past the self-blame that is so characteristic of victims of sexual abuse. The authors of one study assert that most of the victims of professional exploitation whom they see in therapy expressed shame and guilt about the experience (Luepker and Retsch-Bogart, 1986).

Luepker's empirical study shows that 87 percent of her sample blamed themselves for the professional sexual misconduct (Luepker, 1999). As one victim put it: "Yes, he did horrible things. But what about my role in it? On some level—even if it was subconscious, I let him do it. I allowed myself to be his victim. . . . I had colluded in my own victimization. His crime had many names. . . . But I was guilty too, guilty of being his accessory by allowing myself to be his victim" (Noel with Watterson, 1992: 210). What is remarkable about this particular case is that despite a feeling of being both victim and accessory, this woman *did* claim, both in civil court and to remove her exploiter from practice. It is apparent that it is not necessary to absolve oneself from personal responsibility to become transformed into a claimant. In fact, some women seem to have an existential need to hold onto their sense of responsibility for what happened because they feel that otherwise they could not protect themselves in future instances (Luepker, 1989: 192). This may help to explain why Noel felt responsible despite the fact that her therapist had provided her with sufficient quantities of sodium amytal that she became addicted. It was while she was unconscious from the drug that he raped her, hardly the kind of participation one usually thinks of as consent.

This self-blame that many women feel is supported by social attitudes in which others blame the victim for what happened to her (Andrews, 1992). "It takes two to tango; she came on to him," is a commonly held view (Fortune, 1996). This is a very common phenomenon in sexual abuse cases, but it is more pronounced in such areas as acquaintance rape and professional sexual exploitation, where the issue of consent is more amorphous (Bohmer, 1991). Bandura asserts that the blame-the-victim phenomenon is connected to the nature of the practices: "When bad practices are well-entrenched, efforts on the part of concerned individuals to halt them by publicizing their destructive effects are more likely to arouse derogation than sympathy for the victims. To acknowledge the inhumanities arouses self-critical reactions if one does nothing about the situation. It is easier to reduce the discomfort by designating the victim as a bad person than to challenge bad practices that are an accepted part of the social order" (Bandura, 1973). Moving away from self-blame is a very important stage in the transformation process because, like other sexual abuse victims, the more a victim of professional misconduct continues to blame herself, the less likely she is to report the abuse (Gunn and Minch, 1988: 39).

When those women who have been sexually involved with professionals do move toward defining themselves as victims and not responsible, they can begin to feel the anger that drives them to action. This anger may be channeled into political activity of various kinds; complaints to professional associations, licensing boards, or the police; or civil lawsuits. The anger provides those victims who do fight back with the energy and determination to face a situation that may be even more debilitating, as extensively described in the rape literature with respect to victims who file complaints in the criminal justice system.

Not all victims are driven to fight back by feelings of anger. For many, getting to the point where they feel anger is a long process that does not necessarily precede the decision to file a complaint or a lawsuit (Luepker, 1993). Since one of the key symptoms of posttraumatic stress disorder is the numbing of feelings, some women do not initially show anger at the perpetrator even when they acknowledge harm and do initiate a lawsuit (Luepker, 1993).

How the situation is to be defined is not a problematic issue for those who have been subjected to "real" rape, which is unambiguously a crime (Estrich, 1987). For victims of other sexual abuse, the definition of the situation is clearly crucial to the acceptance or rejection of the victim status. Frequently, in the case of date rape, for example, the situation is defined by the man involved as one of consensual sex. The man says, while holding her down, "You want it. I know you do, otherwise why would you be in my room?" It is only when the woman rejects that definition and recasts the encounter as one in which she was forced to engage in nonconsensual sex that she can redefine the encounter as rape and take on the status of a rape victim.

For victims of professional sexual misconduct, the situation may also be defined initially by the man. The professional may assure the victim that the sex would "be good for" her or that it would cure her sexual problems. In the case of *Greenberg* v. *McCabe* (453 F.Supp.765 [E.D. Pa.1978]), the therapist told the plaintiff that she had "a lot of sexual hangups." Julie Roy testified in her trial that "Dr. Hartogs said I must be more open about sexual matters, and that a physical relationship was important because if we were going to work on my homosexuality, it was important that I had a relationship with a man" (Freeman and Roy, 1976: 47, 49). One perpetrator convinced his patient that he would teach her "God's love through a fatherly love" (Lewis, 1995: 49). Perhaps the most outrageous assertion on the part of a therapist came from one who told his patient that sexual contact was necessary to cure her cancer (Bass, 1989). Therapists' self-perceptions may also justify the behavior by defining the sexual encounter as beneficial. In a study of how therapists describe their sexual behavior with patients, one said: "When she came in she was very down. . . . I tried to reach her using a sensory approach. I was trying to communicate to her: caring, love, acceptance, compassion and so on" (Pogrebin et al., 1992: 246).

Victims themselves may define the events in a way that prevents them from taking action. Some of them actually fall in love with the professional. As one victim put it: "I called it a relationship. I felt I was in love with him" (*Crossing the Boundaries*, 1992: 11). Walker says of her relationship with her therapist: "I felt he truly loved me. He would always be there; he told me he would be" (Walker and Young, 1986: 72). Another victim said: "I felt complimented. He'd talk about me from the pulpit" (Doro, 1993). In the therapeutic relationship, these feelings arise as a well-documented part of the therapy, known as transference, but it also exists (though not in the same way) in other kinds of professional relationships (Freud, 1958; Firestone and Simon, 1992: 686; Jorgenson and Sutherland, 1992). There is also some evidence in the literature that those professionals who engage in sexual exploitation select victims because they are particularly dependent and vulnerable personalities (see Schoener, 1989b). One therapist even admitted as much. When asked by the victim whether he was afraid that she or another of his victims might someday report his sexual behavior with them, he replied, "I pick my people carefully" (Bass and Foreman, 1989: 18). These vulnerable victims are more likely to define the behavior in a way that prevents them from taking action.

This "naming" is, according to Felstiner et al. (1981), the first and most important stage in the transformation process toward a legal claim. As long as the events are defined as an affair or a relationship, the victim will not select a script for action which enables her to fight back. Constructing a script for fighting back is made more difficult in our society because so many people believe that sexual behavior between a professional and his client, unless actually forced, is consensual, and therefore not legally or administratively actionable.

Many victims of sexual exploitation by professionals never "name" what has happened as a wrong. In their eyes the situation remains what it was when first defined by them or by the professional. The case of Pat Stern, a patient of the same therapist who exploited Evelyn Walker, illustrates how difficult it is for some women to let go of their initial view of the relationship as one of love and trust. Not only was Stern (who attempted suicide several times during therapy and who became pregnant by the therapist, who arranged for her to have an abortion) unwilling to join Walker's suit, but she was so furious that "her beloved therapist" was being "hounded" by Walker that she threatened to kill her (Walker and Young, 1986).

For other victims, long delays in the naming of a grievance prevent them from complaining. Many people take a very long time to seek help following the exploitation. Jan Wohlberg, a victim of professional sexual exploitation who was a cofounder of TELL, a self-help group for victims of professional exploitation, says that most women wait 7 to 10 years before they are willing to disclose their experiences (Wohlberg, 1993). This is because even seeking help requires some distance and perspective (Luepker, 1989). Victims also may take a long time to decide to fight back. The delay may limit the options available to victims. As one victim told me: "Many people decide not to do anything because of the passage of time; they realize now that they were exploited, but think it was twenty years ago, and the guy might be dead" (Sharon, 1993).

A victim reported that it was not for eight years after the relationship took place that her definition of it changed. "At the time I thought of it as an affair." When she became involved with the task force set up by the College of Physicians and Surgeons of Ontario, she began to name the events as sexual abuse. As a result of her involvement with other victims who laid charges she gradually began to see that she could no longer remain silent about what had happened to her, and she, too, filed charges with the college. She has no plans to file a civil suit against her therapist (Terry, 1993). Any attempt to do so would be fraught with difficulty because of the lapse of time since the exploitation. Many of the civil suits that are filed, even when the delay in naming has not been as long as in this case, revolve around statute of limitations issues.

While some victims gradually come to the realization that they have been sexually exploited, for others, something external triggers their realization. For example, one woman told me: "I was assembling articles for a professor and came across one about confidentiality in reporting. I said to myself 'this is what happened to me'" (Sharon, 1993). Since professional sexual misconduct has recently been the subject of media publicity, some victims first "name" their injury as a result of reading or hearing about other cases. Those who are involved in lawsuits against professionals frequently find that a newspaper article about the lawsuit that gives the name of the professional results in several other women coming forward to claim that they, too, have been exploited by that person.

Some victims do not themselves name their exploitation as such but rather have it named for them by others. Whereas in the case of acquaintance rape victims, this redefinition often comes from friends or parents (Bohmer and Parrot, 1993), in the case of professional sexual misconduct, it may also come from a professional whom the victim subsequently consults. Victims often seek out further therapy to deal with both the original presenting problem and the negative effects of the exploitation itself (Gartrell et al., 1987; Kuchan, 1989).

Publicity about the existence of support groups can also be a factor in the naming process. When a victim first learns of the support group's existence, she may not be sure whether what happened to her "qualifies" as sexual exploitation. If she decides to contact the group, other members, already more sophisticated on the subject, can serve as naming agents for her. They can help her move from self-blame or a feeling of "love" for her therapist to a recognition that the events were exploitation. "'The women of TELL just kept saying that it wasn't my fault, that it was his responsibility. That helped.'" For that woman, meeting another woman who had been abused by the same therapist was also important " 'Until then . . . I still held on to the belief that he really loved me' " (Disch and Wohlberg, 1995: 70). The reluctance to tell anyone about the exploitation is characteristic of these victims. Luepker reports that 96 percent of her sample were reluctant to tell persons close to them (Luepker, 1999). If a victim never tells anyone else what happened, she can hardly move on in the transformation process.

It is not enough for others to define the abuse as such. Victims need to go through the other stages of the transformation process before a dispute becomes a legal grievance, whether in court or before a professional licensing or ethics board. Victims often need considerable assistance in filing charges, as they are unaware of the procedures involved. Many therapists are also ignorant of these procedures or are unwilling either to make the complaint themselves or to provide the support for the victim to make a complaint (Gartrell et al., 1987).

Blaming: Responsibility for the Wrong

The second stage of the transformation process described by Felstiner and his colleagues (1981) is that of blaming. Here the victim, having defined the events as injurious, then focuses on someone else who is seen as responsible for the injury. This stage is more complex here than in most cases because of the relationship that exists between the professional and the victim. It is a much bigger transition from an extremely positive feeling toward a therapist or professional adviser to blaming him than the one in which one moves from a formerly neutral position to one of blame.

Campus sexual assault victims who sue the institution where the assault took place provide an illustrative comparison (Bohmer and Parrot, 1993). When the campus sexual assault victim first "names" the event and defines herself as a victim, she initially blames her assailant. *He* is the person who has caused her the harm, and it is on him that she focuses her fear and, later, anger. After she reports the assault to the campus authorities, the victim becomes involved in the campus judicial hearing process. The members of the college with whom she interacts are initially seen as supportive helpers whose business is to counsel her and to see that the judicial process is properly conducted so that her assailant can be punished for his behavior. At a certain point, however, she begins to recognize that the staff may be protecting interests other than hers and that the college is not as benign as she had originally perceived it to be.

Coming to blame the institution may be a long process, because the victim needs to undergo an about-face in her view of the institution from her initial positive view. The decision to choose this particular college may have been the first major decision the victim has made in her life, usually after long deliberation and discussion. The victim has an investment in the "rightness" of that decision so her initial view of the college is as a wonderful place that can do no wrong.

Similarly, a victim of misconduct by a professional has chosen to place her trust in him. While the decision may not seem as major as the choice of a college, it is, nevertheless, a serious and difficult choice. The seriousness of the choice may depend on the kind of professional chosen; one is likely to weigh more heavily (or at least differently) the choice of a therapist than a lawyer, for example, because of the strong need for trust in a relationship that is based on personal revelation. In both cases, however, the victim begins to rely on the professional as the relationship proceeds. She may see him as very powerful, "godlike," and one who can do no wrong. Roy describes her situation in these terms: "Today . . . she would take the witness stand to give testimony against a man she had once considered only slightly less than a god" (Freeman and Roy, 1976: 1). Once having developed this strong level of trust and even love for the professional, the victim has a great deal of difficulty in coming to accept that he might be to blame for the sexual behavior in which they are involved, as well as its negative consequences.

For victims of campus sexual assault it is easy to ignore or deny the first signs that the authorities are not acting in her best interests, out of loyalty to the institution. Any ambiguity will initially be interpreted to show the institution in a benign light. When a campus sexual assault victim first realizes that the institution also has interests other than her own, she moves from a positive view of its actions to one that is more mixed, in which some of the people she encounters are seen as benign and others malign. Gradually, this process comes full circle to a point at which she moves beyond individual judgments of the members of the college community to a global view of the whole institution as malign. Then the blaming process is complete, and she can move on to the next stage of the transformation process.

Sexual misconduct victims, similarly, spoke of initially believing that the therapist had, indeed, initiated a sexual relationship to help the victim with "her intimacy problem" or her "lesbian tendencies" (Freeman and Roy 1976: 49; *Task Force*, 1991: 65). They also usually miss early cues that the sexual relationship is harmful and negative to them. Instead, as we have seen, they view it as a sign of love or caring. One victim who testified at hearings in Ontario said she thought her social worker therapist really cared about her and was really grateful to have someone treat her as "special" and care about her (*Task Force*, 1991: 65). When the professional engages in other boundary violations by seeing her outside the office or assigning various tasks to her, she sees this as further evidence that she is especially loved and favored. In one case, the victim was seeing a pediatrician for her anorexia. He asked her to baby-sit and engaged in sex with her in his home. She saw this as evidence of how much he needed her. "He was the most important person in my life" (*Crossing the Boundaries*, 1992: Appendix A, 24).

Only later, looking back, can victims see how the pattern of destructive behavior began and what it meant. "After the fact, of course, the unethical nature of his conduct seemed obvious, and I felt ashamed of my obliviousness, mortified at how I had been able to explain away these obvious indicators of impropriety and abuse. It seemed any 'normal' person would have suspected something extremely odd was going on" (Noel with Watterson, 1992: 16). Noel was the victim described earlier who was treated with sodium amytal in excessive quantities over a long period by her therapist, who had sexual intercourse with her while she was unconscious from the drug.

Many victims report that, in fact, they did have "gut" feelings that their sexual relationship with the professional was "wrong" but that they "did not trust" these feelings (Luepker, 1989). Again, it is often much later that they are able to recognize the correctness of their initial feelings and move to blaming the professional for his behavior. Part of the problem with recognizing the "wrongness" of the behavior has to do with the fact that, in many cases, the sexual exploitation is just one part of a series of boundary violations. Luepker reports, for example, that 38 percent of exploiting professionals made unwelcome sexual jokes or comments and that 36 percent asked respondents to perform personal services for them (Luepker, 1999). Those victims who are not sophisticated consumers of therapy do not know that such behavior is also unethical. For them it may be perceived as part of the development of a "special" relationship.

Like the campus sexual assault victims described earlier, victims of professional sexual misconduct may also undergo an about-face in their view of the institution with which the professional is affiliated. For example, it is very difficult for a victim to come to believe that the church to which she has strong emotional ties can have interests other than her protection. Victims often ask: "[H]ow can the Archdiocese or Synod or Church Council be told and then not remove the pastor?" (Luepker, 1993). Ultimately, however, when they have finally come to see that the institution was more concerned with protecting itself and the professional than the victim, they blame the institution as much or more than the professional himself. This is especially true in those cases in which it becomes clear that the church or the licensing board knew of the professional's behavior but, nevertheless, allowed him to continue to practice (Berry, 1992). Many of the victims of clergy sexual misconduct feel obliged to leave the church (Fortune, 1995).

For sexual misconduct victims, the blaming process itself is complex. Blame whom and for what? In many cases, as mentioned earlier, the victim first has to move from blaming herself and accepting the blame of others, to blaming the professional or a third party. For some victims, the professional is blamed for causing further psychological damage either as a result of the sexual relationship itself, which has caused a deterioration in her psychological state, or as a result of the drugs prescribed during the sexual exploitation to facilitate the dependence on the therapist. But for others, the blame may also be because the professional discontinued the sexual relationship. For Evelyn Walker, the anger that usually precedes the blaming part of the transformation process came very late. At a hearing of the Ethics Board of the San Diego Psychoanalytic Institute more than two years after her therapist had discontinued treatment, she said: "I have never been really angry at Zane [her therapist]. I have been hurt and I have been greatly disappointed. It's hard to be angry"(Walker and Young, 1986: 217). Later, during the same hearing, she said: "I don't know that I have ever thought in terms of 'I have been wronged' " (219).

Claiming: Fighting Back through Legal and Administrative Action

For most people, the blaming precipitates the next stage of the transformation process: framing the dispute in such a way as to initiate a claim. A victim usually needs to say, "I have been harmed by this particular person" before she can move on to define the parameters of that harm in broadly legal terms, that of a "case."

Walker's case, described earlier, illustrates, however, that this is not always necessary. Her case was largely framed by others who defined her as having been harmed and who needed her to make a claim against the therapist. Without her evidence, they would not be able to bring charges against Parzen to have him removed from their institute and have his license removed. Walker's motivation was very different; she initially saw her behavior as helping her beloved therapist and, later, as preventing Parzen from harming others. This latter concern arose well into the various hearings that were held and came about only when she found out that several of his previous patients had committed suicide (Walker and Young, 1986). It is a very common motivator for those women who ultimately take action. Roberts-Henry (1995a) reports the results of a survey: "Top priority is preventing abusers from repeating their behavior" (347).

Her decision to file a legal claim also illustrates the significance of the "audience" of external actors in making the decision (May and Stengel, 1990). "When this lawsuit came up, it took a lot of talking of other people to convince me. I weighed this thing very heavily, because I recognized that if I did this, I was starting—there was no choice. . . . I didn't know until he confessed about the other women. I didn't [know] about the dead ones in Chicago. I couldn't ignore it anymore. I had to do something. I had to. And I—I did what I was advised to do by people I trusted" (Walker and Young, 1986: 319). The callers in the British Columbia study reported that of those who spoke about the events with someone else (75 percent of the total), 35 percent of those to whom they spoke suggested that the caller report the experience, although only 2 percent actually made the report themselves (*Crossing the Boundaries*, 1992: Appendix A, 29).

The role of third parties in the claiming process also has a more practical aspect. As mentioned earlier, many victims of sexual exploitation do not know that what has happened to them is a violation of the law or professional ethics. Even less do they know how to proceed if they should decide to claim. It is no doubt for this reason that some states (e.g., California) have mandated that a therapist be required to inform the victim how to file a claim to the appropriate licensing board (Schoener, 1989d). This information-providing role is, of course, central to the role of the lawyer in those cases in which the victim obtains legal advice. Unfortunately, it often takes more than one lawyer before a victim can find one who is both knowledgeable in the area and willing to provide the appropriate assistance. One can imagine that many women make it only as far as the first lawyer, who knows nothing about the issue or is unwilling to get involved in a case against a fellow professional. Thus, while the injury has been transformed into a grievance, it does not result in any legal or administrative action.

Support groups and social movements also serve a role at the claiming stage. They are likely to be better informed than the average lawyer about procedures before appropriate licensing boards. They also perform a referral function, directing the victim to appropriate lawyers and therapists as well as presenting a positive example in those victims who are already at various stages of the claiming process. One of the major functions of such support groups as well as the newsletters of social movement organizations is to provide information and support in a victim's construction of a claim (Durkin, 1991). In short, "the impact of meeting with other people usually sets in action a rippling motion. They end up taking action they never thought they would" (Mary, 1993).

The "audience" can have exactly the opposite effect and discourage the victim from claiming. This is a very common phenomenon in campus sexual assault where victims are routinely discouraged from filing charges either at the campus level or with the criminal justice system (Bohmer and Parrot, 1993). It also appears to be common in the case of professional exploitation. "I used to encourage people more, but now I know what agony they go through, now I feel funny to encourage them" (Pagano, 1997b). Also, the subsequent therapist, while encouraging the victim to see the events as injurious, may, nevertheless, discourage the victim from moving from blaming to claiming. The reasons may be different than in the case of campus sexual assault to the extent that officials of the college are protecting the interests of the college rather than the victim. While therapists may be protecting the interests of their colleagues, they may also believe that there are therapeutic reasons not to claim. A therapist might be concerned about the negative effects of the blame-the-victim phenomenon discussed earlier. In one case of clergy exploitation a victim received "some affirmation of her perception that she had been used, and she came to realize that she also had been raped." The therapist helped her with the naming process but also discouraged her from claiming by telling her that

"women in her situation were usually blamed regardless of what they suffered"(Fortune, 1989: 27).

Some therapists believe that the healing process would be impaired by
too much emphasis on filing charges, especially if they have little faith in
the quality of the courts or the hearing board procedures and outcome.
Putting the events behind her may also be the most therapeutic approach
for a victim. "An awful lot of people have recovered to the point where
they never want to talk about it again" (Roberts-Henry, 1993). Research indicates that, in fact, quite the opposite is the case. Empirical research
demonstrates that taking some sort of action was one of the two factors
most frequently found to be helpful by victims (Luepker, 1999).

The therapist may also argue that the need for the plaintiff to prove
emotional damage in a lawsuit is itself in conflict with the healing process
(Fisher, 1993). The logic works as follows: the more damaged she looks in
court, the more money she will receive. So if the patient recovers well from
the exploitation, she is less able to show that the professional sexual exploitation was extremely harmful and will accordingly receive a lower
award.

For those victims who do fight back, the battle itself may be part of the
healing process. For Julie Roy, the lawyers who took the case were "the
only men she had ever known who fought for her, and at no point put her
down" (Freeman and Roy, 1976: 137). Because one of the major aspects of
professional exploitation is the betrayal of trust, the healing process may
be helped when a victim finds trustworthy lawyers and therapists who act
for her rather than against her in her claim. The sense that the lawyer is
fighting "with" them and "alongside" them has special significance for
some because of their having suffered from domination by someone in a
position of power (Luepker, 1993).

The same sense of empowerment and control can also happen when a
subsequent therapist helps the victim pursue other forms of fighting back.
In one case, the victim credited her therapist for helping her engage in a
face-to-face encounter with her abusing therapist, as well as presenting her
case to the regulatory board in such a way that the board's response was
quick and very positive. "It was an affirming experience," she told me
(P. E., 1999).

Fighting back, while it is an option pursued by very few victims of sexual exploitation, can be a very empowering process, especially if the third
parties (lawyers and therapists) involved are supportive. Not surprisingly,
it is more effective if there is a positive outcome (Ford, 1991). Unfortunately, this is often not the case. As we see in Chapter 8, many victims
complain that they were very badly treated by licensing boards, that the
process was long, and that they felt revictimized by it. One victim who
had been involved in several failed efforts to have her therapist punished
said that "it was very disappointing to me. The APA was the last thing. I

am trying to recover from that" (Sharon, 1993). After hearing testimony from many victims over a period of six months, the Ontario Task Force concluded as follows: "With two exceptions, the complainants we met with had found the process to be daunting, devaluing, and retraumatizing" (*Task Force*, 1991: 87). The sense of empowerment felt by most of those who do take action is also evident in victims of campus sexual assault who sued their assailants as well as those who sued the college (Bohmer and Parrot, 1993). It is clearly strongest for those who win, but even those who lose felt that at least they were in control to a much larger extent than those whose involvement is in the criminal court or with licensing authorities. It is a way to move away from the sense of powerlessness that is so central to the posttraumatic stress suffered by a sexual assault victim, toward emotional strength. As Jeffrey Anderson (1996), a lawyer who represents many plaintiffs in cases of clergy sexual misconduct, puts it: "[B]ringing the lawsuit confronts the perpetrator. That is empowerment." The victim can use the court as a forum to make the events public in the hope that she can precipitate social change both in the institution being sued and in others who learn about the suit. As one victim who had been exploited by a clergyman said: "I wanted to move from being a survivor to bearing witness" (Cindy, 1993). For some, winning or losing is not the issue. When asked by the Arizona Board of Behavioral Health Examiners, "How will you feel if you don't win?," Laurel Park (1994) replied, "I've already won. I've called this guy on his behavior. I know the truth and you know the truth."

Most victims who complain say that they do so in order to prevent the professional from continuing his damaging behavior with others (Luepker, 1993). In some of the cases, victims know of others who have been exploited who are unwilling or unable to complain themselves. The research supports this view that many professionals are multiple offenders. One study of psychiatrists documents that one-third had been involved with more than one patient (Gartrell et al., 1986).

For some victims who sue, however, delays and a feeling that they are being carried along by the process rather than controlling it may limit the positive feelings of empowerment. One victim reported that "you get psyched up to be in the room with the perpetrator. For two weeks I can't eat anything. Then you find out nothing is going to happen. It feels like he is in total control" (Doro, 1993). Despite these feelings, this victim pursued her case to the end, unlike another victim who finally told her lawyers that she was fed up with the process and wanted to settle as soon as possible. "Everything you promised would happen did not," she told her lawyers. She told me that she really regretted filing the lawsuit. On the other hand, this victim felt empowered by her claim to the state licensing board, especially because the therapist who exploited her was "part of the old boy network" (Reed, 1993).

Others blame their lawyers for what they perceive as an unsatisfactory outcome. "He took the case with passion, but toward the middle, they just began to lose it, they didn't want to put money into the case. . . . At the end he just didn't want anything to do with the case . . . . then I settled for a small sum. He coerced me into doing things his way. . . . I'm left with bad feelings all the way around (Barbara, 1998).

The effectiveness of each method of fighting back may vary with the particular experience of each victim. In the case of professional sexual misconduct, a criminal charge or a complaint to the licensing board or the church hierarchy may be more effective in publicizing the issues and preventing others from being exploited. A civil suit often ends in a secret settlement with a "gag order" limiting the ability of the victim to make her claim public. Rutter (1989) points out how damaging gag orders are: "These agreements are extremely harmful to the effort to fight against sexual exploitation. Not only do they suppress truth, but they are analogous to an incestuous father buying his daughter a gift in return for her silence about their relationship" (103). They may also parallel the silence initially required of victims during the sexual misconduct. "It's been difficult for me to break the vow of silence regarding the abuse. Jeanne warned me not to tell anyone about our relationship. She said it would mean 'professional suicide' for her. Like my father and the incest, Jeanne made me responsible for keeping the abuses a secret" (Acker, 1995: 47). Social movement organizations take a very strong position on the negative effects of gag orders, and their newsletters offer advice about how to avoid them or violate them, once made. But there have been few legislative efforts to change the practice. Wisconsin has dealt with the issue as it related to revealing information to subsequent therapists and administrative agencies, and there has been some movement for change from other quarters (Weaver, 1991; Pavalon and Alvary, 1991).[2]

Central to the victim's fighting back through any of the methods available to her is that it moves the victim from one whose primary identification is as "victim" to one whose identification is as "plaintiff" or "complainant" or, even more empowering, social change agent, claimant, or crusader. The exploitation has made her define herself as a victim; fighting back liberates her and provides her with a replacement role and a script for positive action. In that sense, an important purpose has been served regardless of the outcome of the case.

CONCLUSION

The process whereby a victim of professional sexual exploitation becomes a claimant is a complex one that is influenced not only by factors that relate to the victim herself but also by factors within our society. Many victims "drop out" at various points in the process. Some never define themselves as victims who are entitled to redress but continue to accept a script that puts them in the role of participant in the sexual encounter. Others may define the events as injurious but are psychologically unable to take the matter further. Some may confront their perpetrator informally for therapeutic purposes. Some may choose to focus solely on individual recovery rather than overt action, an option strongly supported by the social movement organizations. Others are discouraged from taking action by those with whom they interact. Subsequent therapists may tell victims their recovery will be easier if they put it all behind them; lawyers may say they do not have a case; administrators of licensing boards may make the process so user-unfriendly that victims drop any charges they have filed.

Studies cited earlier indicate that professional sexual exploitation is a widespread phenomenon in many professions. We have also seen that it is harmful for the vast majority of victims. Yet the number of victims who go through the entire transformation process and take their complaint to a legal or administrative conclusion is minuscule.

Several factors appear to contribute to the small number of cases carried through to a conclusion. First, these cases involve the classic gender imbalance of the powerful male and the powerless female. In a factual dispute, society tends to believe the powerful male rather than the powerless, dependent female. This imbalance is exacerbated by the fact that the exploiters are members of powerful and prestigious institutions in our society: medical, legal, and religious institutions. We find it easy to believe that they are simply being harassed by needy women who have fantasized the events they describe. To the extent that this view is pervasive in our society, it also affects the willingness of those who are exploited to fight back.

In addition, we lack understanding about the exact nature of the professional relationship with its extensive coercive power. Thus, even if we believe that what the victim describes did indeed happen, we are sufficiently ambivalent about the role of women in sexual encounters to be more likely to believe that the behavior was consensual, especially if it continued over a period of time. We know from well-publicized rape cases that our attitudes toward consent are central to our acceptance of charges of rape. Such attitudes are even more controlling in cases of professional sexual exploitation in which the issue of coercion is a subtle, but central, element.

A further reason victims of professional sexual exploitation have a difficult time fighting back (especially administratively) has to do with our willingness to allow professionals to control the complaint process by policing themselves. As we see in Chapter 8, professional organizations have been reluctant to accept the possibility that a significant number of their members have been engaged in this sort of behavior. This may be changing as professions have begun to articulate standards of behavior with clients in which sexual behavior is increasingly being declared to be always unethical and sometimes illegal (Bisbing et al., 1995; Jorgenson, Randles, and Strasburger, 1991).

The fact that fighting back is so difficult and relatively rare on an individual level is itself an indication of the lack of success of professional sexual misconduct as a social movement. Given the evidence from incidence research, it is clear that those women whose behavior has been the subject of this chapter represent the tip of the iceberg of the group who has been sexually exploited by professionals. However, as we have seen, it is difficult to measure success in this case. As we see in the case of the support groups, perceptions of success depend very much on how the issue is framed and the expectations the individual has of the consequences of her behavior. Once a victim has taken public action, she is very likely to view the outcome of that action as worthwhile.

In framing any public action as successful, victims are strongly supported by the social movement organizations and the professionals who work with victims. For them, any public behavior is seen in positive terms. As we have seen in the chapter on the organizations, bringing a lawsuit is seen as one of several possible responses, all of which are framed as successful.

As Jeffrey Anderson (1996), a leading plaintiff's lawyer, put it, "[I]f they have found their way to my office, they have made some progress. Usually they have made baby steps; the lawyer is the first or second person they have told." Public action is seen as empowering: "[B]ringing the lawsuit confronts the perpetrator. That is empowerment" (Anderson, 1996). Thus, the action is framed as successful, whatever the outcome. Even if one loses in court, the effort is framed as a success, because one has "broken the silence" and "confronted the perpetrator."

Those involved in the field are careful to make the connections between individual action and the social movement. Confronting the perpetrator is seen both as personally helpful and also as beneficial to the social movement. "Through exposure comes a measure of prevention; the perpetrator risks more if he does something again" (Anderson, 1996). This "prevention" is central to the framing of any legal outcome as a success. Even if one has not been able to punish the perpetrator or his institution through the pocketbook or through loss of his career, one has at least put him and the institution on notice that such behavior is dangerous and potentially costly. As Marie Fortune (1996), a leading spokesperson on clergy sexual abuse said, "[P]rogress is the result of the courage of those of you who have come forward. . . . You have called the Church to be the Church, you have been the Church when it failed to be the Church."

The deterrent value of bringing a lawsuit is also emphasized by those involved in framing the issue. The negative publicity can be effective whether the victim wins in court or not. It affects the reputation of the individual and the institution and alerts other potential perpetrators and victims to the risks of abuse. Thus, for most victims who take action, a number of forces push in the direction of framing their action as a success. This serves to counteract the very real difficulties imposed by the legal and regulatory systems that may result in framing the action as a failure. As we see in the chapters on law and regulation, taking action frequently does not result in what might be objectively measured as success: a verdict for the plaintiff or a strong punishment by a regulatory agency. Fighting back can, however, be viewed as a success as long as a broader definition of success is adopted.

NOTES

1. For the sake of simplicity, I use the term "victim" in its nonpejorative sense.
2. Wis. Stat. Ann. s.895.70(5).

—4—

THE SUPPORT GROUPS

INTRODUCTION

One of the windows through which we can learn about the professional sexual misconduct movement is an examination of the self-help groups that have been formed to provide support and information to victims. Women are frequent users of self-help groups as a way of coping with a wide variety of life's difficulties.[1] These self-help groups for victims of professional sexual misconduct are part of an enormous proliferation of self-help groups in the United States (Powell, 1987). Not surprisingly, this phenomenon has spawned an extensive literature on the subject. Much of it is in the advocacy genre; it describes the self-help movement in glowing terms. Some of the work deals specifically with the experiences of those who have set up various self-help and support groups and advises others how to do so (e.g., Katz et al., 1992). Another part of the literature describes the relationship between professionals and self-help groups and focuses on maximizing the benefits of that relationship (e.g., Powell, 1987, 1990).

Relatively little of the literature is devoted to an examination of the success or failure of self-help groups. In fact, the terms "success" and "failure" are hardly used. We appear to be especially reluctant to examine the possibility that self-help groups, which seem so beneficial in principle to the average person, could be less than an unmitigated success. This chapter examines the role of the self-help group in professional sexual misconduct and the meanings of failure and success in these groups.

The literature that does deal (for the most part indirectly) with success and failure is usually framed in one of three ways: case studies of individual groups, including those that are functioning well (e.g., Barron et al., 1984; Wollert et al., 1982; Harris, 1992), an ecological examination of groups that documents the birth and death of self-help groups (Maton et al., 1989), or an evaluation of the extent to which a group meets the needs of its members as assessed in terms of a variety of traditional measures (e.g., adjustment, rates of hospitalization: see Powell, 1987).

While all of these methods provide partial information about important issues of success and failure in self-help groups, each of them has its own limitations. Single-case studies suffer from the obvious limitation of generalizability. The ecological literature oversimplifies the nature of groups by defining them only in dichotomous terms, as either existing or not existing. Evaluations of the benefits of a self-help group to individual members assume the existence of a vibrant group and use only limited measures of success.

This chapter makes three specific points about success and failure of self-help groups for victims of professional sexual exploitation.[2] First, by the definition of "success" implied in the literature, none of these groups can be considered successful. Second, at least in this type of group, success or failure cannot be defined using only birth and death of the group, as is the case in the ecological literature. Groups do not just exist or not exist as dichotomous categories but rather can be placed on a continuum of functioning, which does not remain constant over the life of the group. To extend the metaphor of birth and death used in the ecological literature, some groups are stillborn, and others are born and live for a short while in frail health, while others live longer, either in robust health or with continuing problems. Third, members of these groups construct the meaning of success or failure in ways that favor success rather than failure. Their conclusions may be different from those that researchers, using "objective" measures, might draw. The knowledge that different people perceive and interpret different events differently is well known and discussed by scholars in several disciplines (e.g., Borkman, 1990; Spector and Kitsuse, 1977; Kahneman and Tversky, 1979). It has also been recognized that "(s)uccess and failure are slippery concepts, often highly subjective and reflective of an individual's goals, perception of need, and perhaps even psychological disposition toward life" (Ingram and Mann, 1980: 12). These insights do not yet appear to have been applied to definitions of success or failure of self-help groups.

Feminist critics of self-help groups argue that the support provided is very personal and emotional (Kaminer, 1992). This, they believe, simply has the effect of making the women members feel better about themselves and their situation, rather than encouraging them to engage in activism to change the system of gender inequality. Taylor's (1996) study of postpartum support groups shows that in that case women do use the groups to redefine the problem and as a basis for activism. As we shall see, such is not the case in the groups for victims of professional sexual misconduct. While a few members have engaged in activism of various kinds, the vast majority do not, and virtually none of it is done as a group.

THE RELATIVE FAILURE OF PROFESSIONAL SEXUAL EXPLOITATION GROUPS

As mentioned before, the literature about self-help groups does not specify a definition of success beyond the ecological one; however, one is implied in the case studies of well-functioning groups (e.g., Katz, 1993: 45; Harris, 1992). Implied marks of success include extensive membership, a number of branches, professional cooperation, a financial base, government and professional action to deal with the problem, and regular, well-attended meetings providing benefits and information to the members. These measures may be more in the nature of ideal types rather than typical of many groups, though the literature does describe some such groups (e.g., Harris, 1992).

When one applies these criteria to the groups for victims of professional sexual exploitation, none of them can be described as successful. This is, in part, a result of choices made by those setting up such groups who decided that their particular members would be harmed by those very things that are seen as a measure of success in the literature. The ways in which the groups for victims of professional sexual exploitation fall short of the implied definition of a well-functioning group are described later.

Characteristics of Professional Sexual Exploitation Groups

The groups for those who have been sexually exploited by professionals frame the issue in rather elastic terms in an effort to broaden their appeal. Survivor Connections uses the definition of "people sexually abused by any type of perpetrator, whether the abuse was done to a child or an adult; and for pro-survivors (defined as supportive relatives, friends or significant others of survivors)" (*Survivor Activist* 2.4, 1994: 1). What is important about this definition and others used by other groups is that no external verification is required. As long as a person says that she has been exploited, she is acceptable as a member of the group.[3] No one is turned away because her exploitation is considered too minor or of the wrong kind. Some groups include among their members those who claim they have been emotionally as well as sexually exploited, those who were exploited as children, those whose sexual exploitation was less than sexual intercourse, those who were exploited by people other than professionals, and partners of those exploited. In addition, there is no limit on how long ago the exploitation took place. A remarkable number of those I interviewed, including some of the most active leaders, had been exploited as long as 20 or even 30 years previously.

These groups do not always have regular, well-attended meetings and an extensive membership. In fact, they have difficulty maintaining membership. Many organizers spoke of having a number of people who came once but never returned; of people finding the group too hard to take; of those who felt that after a few meetings they needed to move on. It is, at least in part, to increase membership that groups are willing to use the broadest definition of professional sexual exploitation.

Professional sexual misconduct groups are not usually part of a larger network of groups with a central organization that provides support and guidance, which is one of the measures associated with survival in the ecological literature (Maton et al., 1989). To the contrary, some leaders express a preference not to be a branch of a wider organization.

These groups are not well financed and operate with virtually no money. They usually survive on what the members provide when the hat is passed around. Additional expenses are met by the person who is committed to the activity, like running the telephone hot line or producing a brochure. This penury is usually intentional; it is related to their reluctance to incorporate, which would be necessary to raise funds. Leaders fear that the more organized they are, the greater the risks for their members from the legal system and elsewhere. But the lack of any financial backing limits what the group can do and may make it more difficult to sustain. It also causes resentment on the part of those members who are footing the bill toward those who are not.

Groups organized around professional sexual exploitation seem to be unable to live with professional leaders but unable to live without them. Professional leaders may represent the "enemy," that is, the professional who was responsible for the exploitation, who is not, therefore, to be trusted. Advice given by professionals who are not involved with the running of the groups may be unwelcome for the same reason. Thus, the groups usually choose to operate without professional leaders. The founders of the group have the momentum to keep the group running for a period of time, but they often suffer burnout and want to hand over the reins to someone else. Sometimes there is no one else as capable or as committed, and the group gradually unravels after the departure of the original leader (Roberts, 1993). Roberts (1993) told me: "The group exists as far as I am willing to work on it." If it does not collapse altogether without a leader, the group may deteriorate into a battle for control among several members (Wohlberg, "Healing," 1993).

The groups often have difficulty finding a suitable place to meet. Without money, many public spaces are unavailable. The church basement, the perfect home for many self-help groups, is unlikely to be acceptable to groups that include people who were exploited by the clergy. Some groups meet in private homes but often find it too big a burden on the homeowner.

Individual group members have made some efforts to push for recognition of professional sexual exploitation as a problem meriting governmental and professional attention, but these efforts have been sporadic and of mixed success, as we see in later chapters. For example, a few members were successful in their lobbying efforts to have professional sexual exploitation criminalized (Roberts-Henry, 1995b; Alexander, 1993b), though others have failed in such efforts (Pagano, 1997b). In general, activism is not a theme of the groups.

The groups have been most successful in the task of providing information and support to their members. That role was mentioned by many of the interviewees as one of the most important benefits of such groups; however, some provision of information and support takes place outside meetings, on the telephone, or at lunch on a one-to-one basis. The group cannot therefore claim sole credit for these activities.

THE CONTINUUM OF FUNCTIONING

Even though none of the groups for victims of professional sexual exploitation can be considered "well functioning," there is a wide range among groups as to how well or badly they are functioning. Some groups are actively functioning, while others either never got off the ground or have not lasted. All groups, including the most active, have undergone changes over the years. The following case studies describe several groups selected to represent different points on this continuum of functioning.

The High End of the Continuum

TELL: Boston

The group most often mentioned as a success among those who work with victims of professional sexual exploitation is TELL (Therapy Exploitation Link Line) in Boston. That group was started in 1989 by several women who had been exploited in therapy who came together through publicity about cases involving two well-known psychiatrists in the Boston area (*TELL Starterkit*, 1993). The group began with about 12 women, and before long attendance rose to over 40 women. The meetings provided opportunities for women to share their stories of what had happened to them and to obtain information about possible legal action and filing complaints with ethics and licensing boards. This information was provided by a lawyer who attended the meetings. A therapist was also invited to a few of the meetings "to lend support" (*TELL Starterkit*, 1993: 6). In addition to meeting monthly, TELL established a telephone line that victims can call for information or support. TELL has played a prominent role over the last several years in efforts to enact tougher legislation in Massachusetts, as well as appearing on television and radio and giving interviews to the newspapers, as part of its education effort. In 1992 the

American Psychiatric Association awarded TELL the Assembly Speakers Award for its contribution to the field of mental health.

That is the successful part of the story: the group satisfied a pressing need; the membership rose; the group received a lot of publicity; and it was recognized by a professional organization concerned with the problem. But unlike other types of self-help groups, it has not been able to duplicate its success by setting up branches elsewhere.

Nor has it become financially successful. TELL does not collect dues and has not incorporated. In fact, it intentionally has very little formal structure; it keeps no membership lists and has no board of directors and no official officeholders. TELL sees structure as increasing the risk that the existence of its group will have a negative impact on those women who take legal action and are required to testify about something that happened in the group (Hoffman, 1994; Wohlberg, "Healing," 1993).

Because it refuses to incorporate, it cannot solicit grants, as so many self-help groups do. Without outside funding, it is the ultimate shoestring operation, doing no more fund-raising than passing the hat at meetings. Without outside funding, it cannot hire even the most modest administrative assistance or pay for advertising to increase membership. The telephone line, which until the development of its Web site was the centerpiece of the organization, was in the home of one of the founders (paid for by her), who responded to all the calls personally on a voluntary basis at considerable personal sacrifice. Now that the group has the Web site, it no longer uses the hot line, thereby reducing the financial and time-consuming burden that previously fell on one member. All TELL's material, including the *Starterkit*, developed to help others start groups, is produced by volunteers at the expense of those who undertake the activity.

TELL began by meeting in private homes and later moved to a church. As a result of the move, the attendance has fallen off, because some women feel less safe in a public place (Wohlberg, "Healing," 1993). It does not advertise where it meets. It tries to do some gatekeeping by assessing at the first telephone contact or in communication over the Internet whether the caller is someone who could benefit from the group or is someone unsuitable for membership. If the caller is suitable, she is advised of the time and location of meetings. TELL still meets regularly each month, though its attendance has fallen off to between 8 and 12 women each meeting. "There is an unending supply of victims," but very few attend meetings regularly (Pagano, 1997b).

TELL has addressed the problem of leadership by having a committee in which each member rotates as leader. Members of this committee are already well into the recovery process, so they are better able to put aside their needs to attend to those of other members of the group. That way, they avoid the difficulties inherent in leaderless groups (no focus, no organization, no control of potential factions) and single-leader groups (resentment about what may be seen as the attempt to garner power, inability of the leader to be able to work on her own issues). With a rotating leader, the decision-making power is diffused, and so is the anger (Wohlberg, "Healing," 1993).

Even with its careful control of leadership issues, TELL has had to change the way the meetings are conducted. Initially, a psychologist was part of the group, but after about a year she was pushed out because she was seen as one of "them," that is, a representative of the exploiters. Initially, the group did not have any formal agenda, but more recently the organizers have come to believe that they needed a more formal approach so that the meetings do not get bogged down in endless repetition of each member's story. As a result, the current format followed is one in which every other month the group has a meeting about a specific topic after a short informal session, and on the alternate months, it brings in an outside speaker to discuss a relevant subject.

Those members of TELL whom I interviewed all stressed that the meetings represented only part of the importance of their group. Much of the activity that they see as important used to go on over the telephone when people first called the TELL phone number and now takes place over the Internet. "People want someone to listen to them. They don't necessarily want to come to a meeting" (Pagano, 1993). Some of those calls were from men who are the "saddest of all. No one takes any notice of them" (Pagano, 1993). Networking between meetings is also seen as crucial: "We make sure that everyone has someone else's telephone number" (Wohlberg, "Healing," 1993).

What is remarkable about TELL are the dedication with which the original founders continue to devote themselves to this issue and their sophisticated understanding of what is needed to keep the group viable. Until recently, the leaders had not cycled out of it, as is so often the case, and two or three of them continued to attend the meetings regularly. Recently, however, one moved away, and another no longer participates in the activities. The success of this group is, nevertheless, strongly tied to the expertise and dedication of the leaders. While not unique, this dedication is remarkable because many victims of professional sexual exploitation are eager to put their exploitation behind them as soon as possible and then have nothing further to do with a group.

The Linkup Group: Chicago

Linkup, the organization for survivors of clergy sexual abuse, which we discuss in detail in the next chapter, has run a support group in Chicago since 1991 for those who have been exploited by the clergy. It meets once a month in a mental health center and usually has an attendance of five or six members. Atypically for these groups, members are mostly male, though one of the leaders of the organization, a woman, is usually the facilitator at the meetings. The group does not have a structure or a specific agenda, but generally the members "go around the table, talk about our own personal issues, discuss all the current dirt going on in the Church. It's almost like a family gathering, a bunch of survivors" (Rick, 1997). The groups sometimes socialize together and keep in touch with each other by phone. The only requirement for membership is that they are survivors or spouses of survivors. All the members of the group are Catholic, and they were all abused by priests as children or adolescents. They believe that they would quickly weed out someone who would be disruptive. They do some initial screening in the first telephone contact, though it is not very specific.

The Low End of the Continuum

Nonstarter: Norfolk, Virginia

When Victoria Cudahy (1993) decided to start a self-help group, she initially spoke to a group called RESPONSE, which provides sexual assault support services in Norfolk, Virginia, but was unable to set up anything through them. She also contacted the Western Massachusetts chapter of TELL for suggestions. She has since been networking in an effort to gather enough women to start a group, so far without success. She has put together a brochure and a bibliography and has spoken at a RESPONSE conference. From that conference only three people expressed interest, insufficient to start a group. She has been trying to work with another victim, but "we couldn't seem to get our schedules together" (Cudahy, 1993). She has tried to persuade three different people from the local newspaper to print an article, but they all felt that the paper had done enough on the subject. She is now trying again to work through RESPONSE so it can help her get started.

Been and Gone: New Jersey

When Kathy Devlin (1999) was exploited during therapy, she felt really isolated and very guilty and depressed. She looked into the possibility of joining a support group but found that none existed, so she started one of her own. She contacted the New Jersey Self-Help Clearinghouse and was trained in how to set up a support group. Devlin put out flyers and obtained members by word of mouth. Most of the time, the group had four members, with a high of six, and some of them "were in really bad shape." They met weekly for a while. They had an informal agenda and tried to keep the focus on empowerment. As time went on, the group became more therapeutic, and some members didn't want it to be that way, so they disbanded after five or six months. There was also some disagreement about goals: "I wanted to do more advocacy . . . the other people didn't want that."

Barely Making It: TERN: Maryland

TERN (Treatment Exploitation Recovery Network) has been functioning since 1992, with a two-year hiatus recently. Most of those involved have also been part of the state task force, which has been very active in examining professional sexual misconduct in the state (see Chapter 8). Some of the task force recommendations have been implemented in law and policy changes, making this group unique in its activist connection, as well as the success of those efforts. The group was started by Cathy Nugent, a professional consultant and educator in this area and one of the authors of the Task Force Report ("Sexual Exploitation: Strategies for Prevention and Intervention," 1996). When the group first started, it was more active; membership ranged from 3 to 11; and it was led by Cathy Nugent, who is no longer involved. The group currently meets once a month at a sexual assault center. If all the members attended, there would be 6 people, but usually there are only 1 or 2 people present, hardly enough to have much of a meeting. It has "been slow getting started" after the hiatus (Russell, 1999). Russell, herself a consumer member of the task force who now runs the group, is hopeful that more members will be referred to the group from the sexual assault center where they meet, which has added sexual exploitation to the brochure listing its services.

EXPLAINING THE DIFFERENTIAL LEVEL OF SUCCESS AMONG THE GROUPS

So, why do some groups work better than others? There are actually two broad types of problems with these support groups. One type of problem is endemic to groups for victims of professional sexual exploitation and accounts for why all such groups have difficulties. The second category of problems is idiosyncratic and affects some groups more than others.

Endemic Problems

The first difficulty encountered in all efforts to start groups in this area has to do with societal ambivalence toward the whole issue of professional sexual exploitation, which is a thread running through this book. Many people, including the survivors themselves, do not see this as a wrong that deserves redress (Bohmer, 1994). For many victims, the predominant feelings are shame and guilt, which are not the kinds of feelings that make it easy for them to join groups and to talk about their exploitation.

Another characteristic of this type of victimization is that, by its very nature, it involves a betrayal of trust. People who are exploited by professionals find it very difficult to trust again, which includes trusting fellow group members and leaders. In one group, for example, the issue of whether to admit men to the group caused great difficulty, which led to the departure of some of the members (Roberts, 1993). Some members who had been exploited by men felt that they could not trust men enough to have them in the group. The only group that is predominantly male is the Linkup group, which is made up of survivors of clergy sexual abuse. The problem with trust is clearly central in the problems with leaders I heard described so often. If a group has a leader, especially a professional, members may fear becoming involved in a repetition of the exploitation that brought them there in the first place. It has led at least one group to decide to get rid of its therapist-leader (Wohlberg, "Healing," 1993).

Another problem characteristic of all groups of victims of professional sexual exploitation stems from the fact that so many group members are seriously psychologically damaged by the exploitation. This damage leads to problems in the group, especially if there is no trained leader who knows how to handle such problems. One of the risks is that the groups will simply become a forum for the eternal retelling of the stories that brought them to the group, without any movement forward. Another difficulty is that the members are all at different stages of recovery from the exploitation. For many of them, their first meeting is also the first time they have talked publicly about what happened. The best situation may be in the Forbidden Zone-California group, where virtually everyone is in therapy outside the group (Haskin, 1993).

Idiosyncratic Problems

One source of problems comes from the fact that, apart from TELL-Boston, none of the groups appear to do any real gatekeeping. Because there is so often a shortage of members and because of the elastic definition of "exploitation," anyone who wants to join can do so. Sometimes, however, a victim may be sufficiently disturbed as to be disruptive or is too early in the recovery process to be able to participate or may not even be a survivor at all (Wohlberg, "Healing," 1993; Hall, 1994). It is much harder to expel members than not to admit them in the first place, with the resulting disruption in the group until that member leaves. Sometimes, instead, the group self-destructs.

Even though these groups allow in anyone who considers herself to have been exploited, comparisons inevitably take place as each survivor tells his or her story. The more successful groups are aware of the risks of such one-upmanship of the "my exploitation was worse than yours" variety and are quick to nip it in the bud (Haskin, 1993). Otherwise, those whose exploitation may not fit the classic version are likely to feel marginalized or further traumatized and leave the group.

The problems of leadership typical of all groups have already been mentioned several times. Unless these groups are managed capably by those who have some understanding of the relevant aspects of group dynamics, they have little chance for success. The best solution seems to be a leader who has some training in group dynamics but who is not seen as a professional, as is the case in CASA (Coalition against Sexual Assault), a group for clergy abuse survivors, where the leader is both a survivor and a trained rape crisis counselor (McLeod, 1994). A further difficulty with leadership is that the founders keep the group running for a period of time but then, as we have seen, suffer burnout and want to hand over the reins to someone else. Sometimes, there is no one else as capable or as committed, and the group gradually unravels after the departure of the original leader (Roberts, 1993).

These groups, as discussed earlier, are the paradigm of volunteer activity. They usually have no money except what the members provide when the hat is passed. Additional expenses are met by the person who is committed to the activity, like running the telephone hot line or Web site or producing a brochure, which can be quite expensive. As we have seen, this penury is usually intentional; only one person I interviewed ever bemoaned the lack of money. But the lack of any financial backing limits what the group can do and may make it more difficult to sustain. It also causes resentment on the part of those members who are footing the bill toward those who are not.

There is a constant need to solicit new members because attrition rates are so high. Some groups started with a pool of members big enough to sustain regular meetings, but as some of those members recovered and moved on, the groups had great difficulty keeping membership up. Several of the people I interviewed spoke of people coming once or twice, seeming to benefit, and then disappearing without explanation. Sometimes external events provide unsolicited and helpful publicity (e.g., the Anita Hill hearings, as well as local cases that get media attention). A group cannot, however, rely on such events without some more regular source of referral. The Forbidden Zone-California group gets referrals from a variety of hot lines that have their number, while TELL-Boston gets referrals from BASTA (Boston Associates to Stop Treatment Abuse), a group of professionals who specialize in professional sexual exploitation, especially the one-day workshops they run. IMPACT (In Motion—People Abused in Counselling and Therapy) in Colorado got referrals from therapists and lawyers (Roberts, 1993). Those who do not have a regular source of referrals are less likely to survive. However, having some members who are "new" and others who have been in the group a long time can itself be a source of friction (Parker, 1997).

Groups that have connections with other organizations generally seem to do better. They can look to another organization to minimize some of the problems mentioned earlier. Some groups are connected with rape crisis organizations, which can serve as a referral source, a location for meetings, and contacts with professionals in the broader field. One national organization, SNAP (Survivors Network of Those Abused by Priests), provides potential group leaders with guidelines for running groups, gives telephone support, and runs weekend sessions to get groups started (Hall, 1994).

Groups need a clear sense of how to deal with their particular safety and confidentiality issues in order to survive. For example, at a meeting of the western Massachusetts TELL, someone slit the tires outside the house where the meeting took place. "No one at that meeting has ever come back" (Yaukey, 1993). It was never determined who did it, but the women were convinced it was directed at them. One person came to the Forbidden Zone recovery group with the intention of writing a book about the members. When the group found out about this, "it shattered" (Parker, 1997). This event caused one of the founders to use a pseudonym and a box number for all related correspondence. Even a message left on a member's telephone machine could cause her to leave the group if other members of her household did not know about the exploitation, and she felt she could no longer trust the other group members.

A final, but important, factor that affects the group's success or lack thereof is, unfortunately, one over which members have no control. The region of the country in which a group exists seems to play an important role in whether it survives or not. It is no accident that the case examples of more successful groups were in Boston and the Bay Area, among the most liberal and heavily populated areas in the country. People are more open and accepting of such groups and the issue that brings members together in those areas than, for example, in the South. In Boston and the Bay Area, there appears to be a more constant flow of publicity about various aspects of the problem that provides a stream of new members to replace those who leave. This seems not to be true elsewhere, as is illustrated in the case of one woman who used to fly from Texas to the Bay Area to attend meetings (fortunately, her husband worked for an airline) (Haskin, 1993). When she stopped commuting, she was unsuccessful in her efforts to set up a group in Texas. Many of those interviewed lived in sparsely populated areas where it simply was not possible to gather together enough victims to make a group.

A PARTIAL SOLUTION: THE WORLD WIDE WEB

The advent of the Internet for communication among survivors of professional sexual misconduct has done much to solve the problems of support groups. Kevin Gourley, a longtime computer professional and the husband of a victim of professional sexual abuse, set up an Internet information service (http://www.advocateweb.com) to provide the information and support he and his wife found to be lacking when they were dealing with her exploitation. It provides links to other relevant Web sites, including TELL's Web site, and links to useful information of various kinds (news stories, information about law and ethics, information about upcoming conferences and retreats, etc.). It has both an e-mail peer group forum and a Web discussion forum for people to communicate with each other. According to Gourley (1999b), the Web site has worked out very well, though he has had to deal with a couple of difficult situations in which people have been able to "take advantage of the anonymity it permits to mislead participants." For example, one person was posting some really bizarre messages that the other participants found very upsetting, and it turned out that she was using different names and actually carrying on a conversation with herself. As a result of this problem, Gourley has turned on a feature on the forum where he can, if absolutely necessary, see the Internet address of the person posting the messages. This is an example of the delicate balance between anonymity, on one hand, and legal and psychological protection (both for the members and for Gourley as Web master), on the other. In an effort to deal with this problem, Gourley has posted quite an extensive set of disclaimers on the e-mail peer support discussion list.

The benefit mentioned most often by those users with whom I communicated is very much the same as that of support group members: being able to talk to someone who "understands." "I find it much easier than talking, and hearing and reading what other people write makes me see that I am not alone in my feelings" (Lisa, 1999). For one user, the Web provided an "unusually vast ability to contact others who have been through—or who are going through the abuse/exploitation process. They understand. (Whereas I cannot get this same feedback from normal family and friends—some cannot even hear me)" (Jan A., 1999).

Concerns about trust exist in the on-line groups just as they do in self-help groups. In some ways concerns about trust are easier to deal with on the Internet, where people can keep their identities secret and need reveal no more about themselves than they wish. By the same token, however, they can misrepresent themselves, as the members are aware. Since the people with whom they communicate do not know who they are, the risks that their secrets would be betrayed are less than in the face-to-face encounters of self-help groups. On the other hand, this privacy is, to some extent, illusory, as many of the participants know. For example, the Web master is concerned about the possibility that the e-mail could be subpoenaed in a court case, just as information in a support group is at risk, but this has not yet happened (Gourley, 1999a). Material is more available for subpoena or other unwanted uses; unlike telephone conversations, which are generally not recorded, there is a record of e-mail.

The issue of trust may be one of perception; some people feel safer with the anonymity, while others fear the risks of people "invading" their e-mail more than they fear the other members of a support group or the person at the other end of a hot line. These fears are all too characteristic of victims of professional sexual exploitation; some participants fear that their abuser might be able "to 'lurk' in the forum thereby causing further harm and re-victimization" (Jan A., 1999). The "terms and conditions" of participation in the peer support discussion lists include a condition that the person is not a professional who has abused someone, which provides protection from legal liability if an abuser lies about his status but could nevertheless cause the harm that participants fear.

One of the great benefits of the Internet is that it is accessible to anyone who has an Internet connection, regardless of where he or she lives. We have seen that support groups are simply not available for those who live in isolated areas or areas where people do not want to talk about the problem, even in a support group. This need to muster enough members and, even more importantly, to keep up a continuous supply is not necessary in the case of communication on the Internet. Support is also available at any time the person feels the need; one user said that "it is a forum to go on 24/7 to read and/or vent about this subject and its related issues" (Jan A., 1999). Some survivors are so filled with self-doubt and shame about the exploitation that they will never be able to seek out a face-to-face support group; for them the Internet provides a lifeline.

For some users, this has been a unique form of support: "Hopetalk is a place where I always find compassion, understanding, and, most importantly, a common bond with others who have the same pain in their soul" (Athena, 1999). Other users see it as a supplement to other sources of support, if they are available, rather than a replacement of them: "I don't think this type of forum should replace face-to-face support groups or therapy, but be an addition to that" (Lisa, 1999). Another said, "The online support group has been a lifeline to me. I take what I learn there back to my individual therapy for examination" (C. D., 1999).

For a group like TELL, operating its Web site can divide the burden of responding to queries more evenly than was the case when the hot line was in the home of one member who was responsible for organizing the responses to the calls. Gourley, the Web master, tells a very similar story to those I heard from people who set up support groups. Despite the extensive help of his wife, Gail, he feels the burden of bearing all the responsibility for the Web site. They have spent an inordinate amount of uncompensated time working on the Web site, first in setting it up and then in managing it. They, too, are trying to work out a way of being compensated for their time, perhaps by becoming a nonprofit organization.

While it is clear that some of the problems of support groups are mirrored on the Internet, others are not. At the very least, it provides a widely available supplement to self-help groups.

CONCLUSION

Success and failure are socially constructed concepts that reflect the needs and interests of those constructing them (Spector and Kitsuse, 1977).

The construction of success and failure has been shown to depend on the frame of reference selected by the person involved. Prospect theory asserts that the way people frame a decision that they make determines, in part, how they see the consequences of their decision. People first pick a reference point and assess outcomes from that reference point (Kahneman and Tversky, 1979).

The decision to try to set up a self-help group can be assessed in light of these concepts. It is framed in terms of the isolation of victims of professional sexual exploitation, which includes the need to talk about what happened with fellow sufferers, the need to understand the normal course of recovery, and the need to obtain information about what legal and administrative action is available. The isolation felt by those women who made efforts to set up groups is caused, in their perceptions, by the tremendous silence that so many people describe as surrounding this problem. Thus, the reference point from which they begin their efforts is this silence and the isolation it causes and the resulting need to do something to reduce it. They have a great need and few expectations. Anything they perceive as reducing their isolation and ignorance about the problem will therefore be viewed by them as successful. Thus, the women I interviewed were very anxious to define their groups as "successful," even if they were no longer functioning or barely functioning and had virtually none of the objective characteristics of a well-run group. While a number of them did express frustration at the limitations of the groups they were involved with, this frustration was played down, and the benefits were played up.

The interviewees all stressed the benefits of any kind of contact with another victim because it showed that other women had had this experience. As one woman said: "You meet another person, it's like looking in a mirror" (Roberts, 1993). One central aspect of the benefit of contact revolves around providing referrals to lawyers and sympathetic therapists, and advice about official ways of responding to the exploitation, including complaints to licensing boards and ethics committees, and filing lawsuits. This can be done outside the group through the Internet, networking, telephone contacts, or brochures on legal options. One woman said that "the best kind of group is a referral and advocacy group. You don't need a group, you can get it on the phone. What I needed was help on my complaint" (Marge, 1994). For this, the Internet is the most useful source of information. It is likely that the need for support groups has diminished somewhat since the Internet has been able to provide both information and interaction with other survivors of professional sexual misconduct, though, as we have seen, some users do not believe that it replaces the personal quality of face-to-face support.

The women I interviewed also define the term "group" in ways very different from its meaning in the literature. Such definition makes possible the perception that the "group" is a success. More than one of the founders of a group consider it still to be a group, though it no longer holds formal meetings (Migliori, 1993; Roberts, 1993). One woman described a "group" that came about as an offshoot of a therapy group in which five women go out for dinner together every month. They have gone skiing together, and two of the women walk together regularly. Another group has developed into a kind of women's art collective in which the making of fabric assemblages is used as healing (Yaukey, 1993). After failing to put together a group among several victims, one woman framed it as a success rather than a failure. She said: "[T]he women are now doing it (interacting) on a one-to-one basis" (Pitt, 1993).

These self-help groups provide an excellent illustration of the centrality of framing for an understanding of the meaning of success and failure. Despite the evidence that all groups for victims of professional sexual exploitation suffer from difficulties both in getting started and in surviving, the way success and failure is framed shows that these groups may nevertheless be defined as successful by their members even if they are not actually functioning or barely functioning. Those who would examine success and failure in "objective" terms present an oversimplified picture of success and failure when applied to self-help groups for victims of professional sexual exploitation.

NOTES

1. Material for this chapter comes from about 40 interviews with women (and one man) who have been actively involved in attempts to set up self-help groups around the country for victims of professional sexual exploitation. Additional material was obtained from in-depth interviews with about 20 professionals who work in the area of professional sexual exploitation, some of these interviews on several occasions. Names of the respondents were obtained through use of a snowball technique, initially from professionals who work in this area and from the section on resources in *Sex in the Forbidden Zone*, Peter Rutter's standard text on the subject (Rutter, 1989). Almost all of the respondents (including victims) were willing to have their names used; those who were not have not been quoted directly, or I have used only first names. None of the respondents were, however, willing to let me participate directly in the groups themselves because of their concern about confidentiality. For that reason, I have had to assume that the information provided by the group organizers and the professionals is an accurate description of the process of setting up and running the groups. For further details of the method used, see Bohmer, 1995a.

2. Much of the current literature has eschewed the term "victim" in favor of the term "survivor" or "victim/survivor" because of what are viewed as the pejorative connotations of the word "victim." I believe that the traditional meaning of the word "victim," one toward whom a negative act has been perpetrated, is not pejorative and is clearer (see Bohmer, 1994 and discussion in Chapter 3). For this reason, I use it here.

3. Since the vast majority of these self-help group members are female, the female pronoun is used.

—5—

ORGANIZATIONS AND THEIR ROLES

INTRODUCTION

The literature on social movements tells us that social movement activity goes on both within formal organizations and elsewhere. Special organizations set up to promote the movements do, however, play a central role in them by creating social movement culture and the development of a collective identity (Johnston and Klandermans, 1995; Taylor and Whittier, 1995). In the case of professional sexual misconduct, most of the social movement activity, albeit limited, is generated by the organizations. These organizations are involved in framing the movement, recruiting members, developing group norms, and providing the setting for the playing out of rituals (Taylor and Whittier, 1995). In this chapter, I examine the organizations and public activities to see what exactly is going on in this social movement, whether it is successful or not, and why.

Before looking at the organizations specifically set up to make claims about professional sexual misconduct, it should be made clear that framing activities are also undertaken by organizations for professionals generally (e.g., the American Psychological Association, American Psychiatric Association, National Association of Social Workers, Clergy Organizations) whose primary role is to represent the profession generally. These organizations, however, are part of the dominant culture and provide a framework consistent with that culture, while the organizations whose purpose is solely that of social movement organizations for professional sexual misconduct are outside the mainstream.

All the professional organizations of the helping professions have developed policies on the unacceptability of sexual contact between patients/clients and professionals. They have discussed the matter at board meetings, held hearings on the subject, produced documents outlining their position, and listened to empirical research on the subject at their professional conferences. All these activities have produced modest media attention outside professional publications and serious attention within those publications. Clergy organizations have also addressed the issue, though in some cases—most notably the Catholic Church—only in response to reports of many claims of clergy sexual abuse. They, too, now have a policy on the subject and continue to address the issue at their meetings and produce statements for the media to publish. The Conference of Bishops has a committee on the subject of sexual abuse by the clergy.

Professional organizations are not, of course, set up to make claims about the nature and extent of professional sexual abuse. To the contrary, they represent the interests of their members, among whom are numbered the perpetrators of professional sexual misconduct. Thus, much of their role here is a defensive one in which the organizations work to play down the seriousness of the issue or to show how well it has already been dealt with by the institutions they represent. For example, while the Catholic Church has on occasion expressed its concern about the charges of sexual abuse by clergy, it attempts to define them as a few bad apples who are being adequately handled within the church. Thus, while acknowledging that a small problem may have existed in the past, it is claimed that it is now solved. Other professional organizations all have firm policies prohibiting professional sexual misconduct but are more and more inclined to leave the policing of violations to other institutions.

The organizations set up specifically to make claims about professional sexual misconduct tell us more about the nature of the social movement. They frame the problem and work to maintain public attention for it. They also work to counter those claims by professional organizations that the issue is not a serious one or that it has already been successfully dealt with. In addition, the organizations encourage people to define themselves as victims/survivors and to engage in individual and group activity to promote the cause.

The organizations that exist in this area primarily cater to those who have been exploited by members of the clergy, though one of them, Survivor Connections, positions itself as an organization for all kinds of professional sexual misconduct as well as all kinds of sexual abuse, while the Linkup deals with all kinds of clergy misconduct. TELL (Therapy Exploitation Link Line), which was discussed at length in the chapter on self-help groups, could perhaps be defined as a network, though it does not put out a newsletter or hold conferences as the other networks do. Another Boston-based organization, BASTA, is a more professional organization. It offers consultation, advocacy, workshops, individual groups, professionally led groups, and training for professionals, all for a fee, rather than as a voluntary organization like the networks described earlier. Apart from TELL, three networks profess to be national in scope:

Survivor Connections, SNAP (Survivors Network of Those Abused by Priests), and the Linkup. More recently, a Web site has been established to provide information and networking to those involved with the issue, with links to other relevant sites, such as TELL and BASTA (http://www. advocateweb.com). Each of these groups was started by a victim or someone close to one. The Linkup was started by the mother of a victim, and the Web site, by the husband. In each case, victims suffered from the absence of information and support that they believed a group could provide and decided to provide them for others. They began as local support groups and then expanded to become national organizations. The groups are atypical of social movement organizations in that none of them have developed out of existing organizations, which Friedman and McAdam (1992) argue is "perhaps the single most successful strategy for launching an SMO" (162).

Interviews with the leaders of the groups indicate that Survivor Connections has 1,500 people who receive their newsletter, SNAP has 3,300, and the Linkup has 7,500, while TELL had over 1,000 participants as of late 1998 (Sara Fitzpatrick, 1995; Clohessy, 1995; Economous, 1997; Wohlberg, 1998). The Web site had .75 million hits in a little over a year, though there are no figures of the number of people who use it (Gourley, 1999a). One cannot, however, use any of these figures as a definitive indication of interest in the issue, as membership numbers can be expected to fluctuate and may have been quoted at their peak. It can also be assumed that there is overlap in those numbers from one network to another, with some people belonging to more than one network.

In addition to the major organizations, a number of other, smaller organizations usually have a specialty focus, as their names indicate, like SMART (Stop Masonic Ritual Abuse Today), New England Patients' Rights Group, Empower the Child, CARAC (Committee against Ritual Abuse of Children), Associates in Education and Prevention in Pastoral Practice, SESAME (Supporters of Educator Sexual Abuse and Misconduct Emerge), CASSANDRA (Supporting, Advocating, Networking, Daring to Recover Association). Some of these groups are very little more than one motivated individual and a newsletter, some are no longer even that, and some have merged with one of the three networks, while others are set up as a base from which professionals can consult and sell their services to others.[1]

The three major networks (Survivor Connections, SNAP, and the Linkup) are generally similar in goals and activities, though they have some regional focus (Survivor Connections is in Rhode Island, the Linkup is based in Chicago, and SNAP is in Chicago and St. Louis). All three have a newsletter, sponsor support groups, give telephone advice to survivors, arrange conferences, and keep a database for survivors to trace their perpetrators and other survivors of that perpetrator. They differ, however, in their emphasis, their political stance, and their success. For example, Survivor Connections is more focused on its database than are the others. SNAP is more independent of church authorities than the Linkup, which is more willing to work directly with the authorities and to accept money from them (Clohessy, 1995). The Linkup is more diverse in the denominations of its members than the others, which mostly cater to those abused by the Catholic Church. SNAP is more involved in personal healing and has a higher proportion of survivors as members than Survivor Connections. Survivor Connections appears to be generally the most outspoken of the three, though the leaders of each group describe their counterparts as more radical than they are! The Linkup appears to be the strongest organization of the three. It is the only one that pays any staff; its president is paid and is therefore able to devote more time to running the organization. The others are dependent on the availability of volunteers and have had periods when they have been moribund. For a period during 1996–1997, Survivor Connections suspended its newsletter for lack of money and people available to put it together. It is currently being published twice a year instead of quarterly as it used to be.

It is interesting to speculate why the organizations focus mostly on clergy sexual abuse, rather than all types of professional sexual misconduct; the reason may be related to the greater ambivalence associated with therapist abuse, which has been discussed earlier. Many of the clergy survivors were abused as children or adolescents, a situation that has less potential stigma and personal responsibility attached. In addition, those abused by the clergy have a more specific target in the church, which they see as responsible for the problem, in addition to the clergy member himself. Those abused by other professionals can blame only the professional.

In addition to the networks and the various other organizations, an important part of the social movement is located in the conferences on the subject, sponsored either by the networks or by a combination of support groups and various professional organizations. The 1998 conference was billed as the Fourth International Conference on Sexual Misconduct by Psychotherapists, Other Health Care Professionals and the Clergy. It was the first of these conferences to tie in misconduct both by the clergy and by other health care professionals; until then, these conferences focused almost exclusively on therapists and other health care professionals, while the conferences sponsored by the networks focused on misconduct by the clergy. Social movement activists are now beginning to develop the collective identity of a more cohesive social movement, rather than a fragmented one, or even *very* small movements.

These conferences provide an important forum for the development of the collective identity of the social movement through networking, the exchange of ideas and information, and the development of norms. The leaders in the field are always present, as are lawyers and therapists, as well as survivors themselves to tell their stories. The mix of each of these groups depends on who is sponsoring the meeting; the networks have more survivors and fewer professionals, while the conferences sponsored by other organizations are more professional. We now turn to several case studies of the organizations and meetings to learn more about the social movement organizations.

SURVIVOR CONNECTIONS: THE CHECKERED CAREER OF A NETWORK

As we have seen, networks provide a central part of the social movement of professional misconduct. This section describes the formation and operation of one of the networks, as well as its decline. As an altar boy, Frank Fitzpatrick was sexually abused by Father James R. Porter. His memories returned to him as an adult, and he embarked on a search for Porter (*Survivor Connections*, n.d.: 1). He describes his "journey" as follows: "I made public speeches—alone at first—for two and a half years; phoned my perpetrator and taped his admission of guilt, put ads in the newspapers to find other survivors, and then appeared with seven other survivors of Porter to break the story on Boston television in May, 1992."

Fitzpatrick started the network in response to calls he received from people looking for support and advice, who had heard about him through his "journey." "They wanted to know how to take action, how to talk about it, where else they could go for help" (1). While the network was originally set up for the victims of Father Porter, the organization now has as its mission the assistance of survivors of all forms of sexual abuse. In fact, the network defends itself vehemently against what it sees as an inaccurate depiction of it as representing only clergy abuse victims or, worse, Catholic bashers, although their own statistics show that the highest number of perpetrators (994) in their database are Catholic priests (*Survivor Activist*, 1998: 6). "One might as well describe us as an organization for green-eyed, left-handed bisexual survivors of sexual abuse by women over 65 years old occurring only on alternate Tuesdays" (*Survivor Activist* 2.4, 1994: 1). The expansion of the frame is here carried out by ridiculing what the network defines as the cultural view of it. They are engaged instead in reworking the frame as one concerned with an important social issue (Swidler, 1986).

The network is run out of the home of Frank Fitzpatrick and his wife, Sara, who describes herself as a survivor of sexual abuse, though apparently not by the clergy (S. Fitzpatrick, 1995). Most of the organizational work is done by Sara and a few volunteers, who help put out the quarterly newsletter sent to about 1,500 people, 900 of whom are survivors, the rest being resource people, ranging from lawyers to therapists to those in other organizations with a similar interest. Subscriptions to the newsletter provide the funding for the network, which is the usual shoestring operation with the usual problems. The Fitzpatricks talk about applying for grants, but no one has so far had the time to do so. The newsletter dated November 1996 informs subscribers that Sara has taken a paying job and will no longer be available to answer calls from survivors. The newsletter was cut to two issues after 1996 instead of the usual four. The newsletter also alludes to its dire need for funds and makes clear that only paid-up members will receive future issues. For a period in 1997, the newsletter was not published for want of funds and personnel but was apparently saved from extinction by an anonymous donation from a New England foundation (*Survivor Activist* 5.2, 1997: 12). Perhaps for the same reason, the network no longer directly sponsors and organizes the To Tell the Truth conferences but instead has "assumed the role of tracking and coordinating these independently-run and locally-managed conferences" (*Survivor Activist*, 1998: 6).

The Fitzpatricks see their major role as providing information about perpetrators, helping victims find their perpetrators, and connecting victims of the same perpetrator to one another. To this end, they have gathered a database of what they describe as "over 3,300" survivors and family members who have called to report that they have been sexually abused[2] (*Survivor Activist*, 1998: 6). "When more and more people speak out . . . [it becomes] a one by one revolution. People speaking out will stop the second victim . . . each survivor needs to speak out until the perpetrator is exposed and brought to justice" (F. Fitzpatrick, 1995). Fitzpatrick is not concerned about educating people, changing social attitudes, or mobilizing for collective action. "I am not concerned about what organizations do. I am just concerned about people speaking out and taking action for themselves and preventing it from happening to others. We are promoting the worship of St. Ayn Rand" (F. Fitzpatrick, 1995).

Fitzpatrick is writing a book on his experience with father Porter, and he also tells his story at a variety of venues ranging from a coffeehouse in Providence, where he performed "unannounced and uninvited," to the fourth international conference in Boston in October 1998 (*Survivor Activist* 5.2, 1997: 11). His performance is a rather strange combination of slides of himself and his family as a child, a description of his molestation, and various songs he wrote on the subject.

THE WEB SITE

The Web site, the most recent of the "organizations" to address professional sexual misconduct, has a history that is remarkably similar to that of the networks and the support groups. It was started by Kevin Gourley, the husband of a woman exploited by a law enforcement officer attached to a special mental health unit. Their "lives were turned upside down," but they suffered the typical difficulties in naming the problem and finding someone who knew anything about it (Gourley, 1999a). As someone who had been involved with computers for over 18 years, it was "very natural for me to turn to the Internet for help and resources." He discovered that there was information available, but it was hard to find, and there was virtually nothing on the Internet. Given his background, it was very natural for Gourley to start a Web site to provide a central place for people to obtain information and "connect with each other and the 'net.'" By then, he had been in touch with the various major players in this field and was able to make himself available to them for any information or resources they wanted to put on the Net.[3] Gourley views the Web site as very successful; it has had .75 million hits, though he cannot give figures of the number of people who use the site. He says that he "sees it impact lives." He has set up a discussion forum that serves the same function as the hot lines operated by TELL and the Linkup. Gourley has also been instrumental in putting together a group of advocates who are available to give advice to those seeking it or to provide information about resources in different areas. He does, however, see a problem, typical of the Web, in the use of the site as a substitute for a support group, as there is none of the screening that goes on, either formally or informally, in support groups. On the Internet "you don't really know who you are talking to. If someone wants to do something (e.g., a perpetrator) it could be harmful. In real life, the person can't come into the room." He also spoke of the relative lack of security of e-mail as a problem for some survivors; unlike the telephone, which is relatively private, e-mail is not.

Like all the other networks and support groups, there is no money to pay for this enterprise. As is typical, Gourley is doing this alone with the help of his wife, spending his own money and time. He worries about its dependence on his experience and willingness to operate the Web site. He does it in his spare time, though he would give up his job "in a heartbeat" if he could figure out some way of supporting himself through it. He is considering his options, whether perhaps to form a tax-exempt corporation or to set up an on-line database with restricted access. He also worries about the legal issues: what to do about suicide threats, whether people can be anonymous, whether to warn people of the risk that material could be subpoenaed. While no one has yet subpoenaed any material, he sees it as a very real risk.

Given the isolation, both physical and emotional, of most victims, the Web site is clearly a tremendous asset as a source of information and help. It is limited by the amount of material that is actually available and the personnel available to keep that material up to date.

MEETINGS

One of the major tools of a social movement is gathering supporters together at conferences and local gatherings. Such meetings serve, among other things, to supplement the information and support available by

telephone and through the newsletters. Both the networks themselves as
well as other groups have held conferences on professional sexual misconduct. The Linkup has had six (as of 1998) annual conferences, which
the organizers say usually draw several hundred survivors and other attendees, though the one I attended in 1997 had only about 100 participants. Survivor Connections has had several conferences, which they also
say drew several hundred people. SNAP has had several regional meetings and one national conference, which drew very few people. Groups
other than the networks have also arranged conferences; for example, the
1994 It's Never O.K. conference was arranged by CHASTEN, a support
group in Toronto, while one held in Fredericton, New Brunswick, was organized by a coalition of health professional groups, and the one in Boston
in 1998 was hosted by the Boston Psychoanalytic Association.

IT'S NEVER O.K.: TORONTO, 1994

This conference, which is fairly typical of all the conferences in its theme
and purpose, was billed as the third international conference on sexual exploitation by health professionals, psychotherapists, and clergy.[4] Its con-
tent was also typical, mostly professionals giving advice and a little
research and also some survivors telling their stories. It was organized by
CHASTEN (Canadian Health Alliance to Stop Therapist Exploitation
Now), the Toronto-based survivors group, which obtained funding and
other support from the Toronto Ministry of Health. It is also typical that
much of the momentum for the survival of CHASTEN was the organization of the conference; as of 1998, it is no longer functioning. The main part
of the conference was opened (which is atypical) by the Ontario minister
of health, Ruth Grier, who in her remarks spoke of the recent legislation
passed in Ontario and lent an aura of respectability and the possibility of
government concern about the subject to the proceedings. She spoke of
"our vast potential to effect change," thereby emphasizing both collective
identity and mobilizing potential.

The mobilizing theme was echoed at many points throughout the conference, with responsibility placed on the shoulders of all present. "Every
single person here has a shared responsibility to create something here
that is useful, effective, and to carry it with us into our work and professional lives" (Firsten, 1994). This responsibility may, perhaps, have been
made easier by the assertion that hundreds of us present were "experts in
the field" and therefore could be expected to bring this expertise to bear
onto the creation of something useful outside of the conference. This expertise can take various forms, the conference was told: "Many of us bring
the expertise of having been a survivor, others bring the expertise of strug-
gling with patients, keeping boundaries, the expertise of those who have
sinned, the expertise of those of us who carry the burden, and share those

of our colleagues" (Firsten, 1994).[5] The importance of nonacademic expertise is a characteristic of all such conferences, even this one, which was among the more professionally dominated of those held on the subject. Everyone had to be seen as an equal member of the mobilizing enterprise, particularly in an issue such as professional sexual exploitation, where power and status differentials are perceived as central to the problem itself.

The twin themes of expecting participants to take something important away from the conference and universal expertise were put into more specifically activist terms by another plenary speaker who saw the group as "fueling our political activism with the raw material of our lives" (Butler, 1994). This speaker placed professional sexual exploitation firmly within the framework of radical feminism, in which it is part of the pattern ranging from stranger rape to marital rape to grandfather and extrafamilial abuse, some of whose victims included the "male survivors of the Catholic Church, white boys in orphanages, brown boys in residential schools" (Butler, 1994).

To Butler, the responsibility was placed firmly on the shoulders of men, for whom, by analogy with James Baldwin's comment on race, "being a man is a moral and ethical choice. Good men don't often take the next step of aligning themselves with us. Instead, they punish the bad men individually without recognizing that there is a more socially constructed expression of masculinity" (Butler, 1994). Thus, the collective identity of the social movement included only those men who constructed their identity in ways acceptable to the movement, which included appropriate activism. Such a radical approach is rather unusual, especially for those activists engaged in extending the framework of the problem to include both male and female survivors.

This conference set about developing a collective identity by borrowing rituals from other groups. For example, the opening reception involved various artistic contributions and a dance recitation portraying "a strong woman." On the second day a woman lit sage and carried it around the room and led a prayer. This ritual, we were told, was called "smudging," a traditional Native American way to begin the day. Such borrowings can be risky if they do not become part of the culture of the social movement. If successful, however, they are an expression of the spillover from one movement to another and provide links among related movements. However, in the subsequent meetings I attended, there was no evidence that these rituals had been taken up as a more permanent theme of the movement.

The international dimensions of professional sexual misconduct were frequently stressed during the conference and highlighted by the involvement of people from several countries, both as participants and presenters. The presentation of research conducted in Australia and New Zealand reinforced the theme that, indeed, this is a worldwide and serious problem. In fact, participants from Australia and New Zealand decided at that conference to mount their own conference, which was held in 1996 in Sydney, Australia.

A SURVIVOR NETWORK CONFERENCE: FIRST INTERNATIONAL MEETING OF SNAP (SURVIVORS NETWORK OF THOSE ABUSED BY PRIESTS): WASHINGTON, D.C., NOVEMBER 1996

Unlike the It's Never O.K. conference, this meeting was directed specifically toward survivors, defined as those abused by *clergy* of any denomination. Virtually all of the survivors present were Catholics abused either as children, adolescents, or adults. The speakers, however, did reflect the broader mission of SNAP by addressing sexual misconduct in all religious denominations. Marie Fortune, one of the leaders of the clergy sexual abuse movement, began her talk with a description of a recent Buddhist retreat for survivors she had been invited to facilitate, to illustrate that the problem reaches even those whose public image would lead one to expect that their priests are not involved in sexual misconduct.

Despite their efforts to cast the net widely, not to mention the rather grandiose billing of the conference as "international," very few people attended. I counted approximately 30 people present. The publicity made it clear that the conference was being held, in part, as a fund-raiser, and the fee of $175 for the weekend was intended to generate funds, had attendance not been so thin. This provides another example of the failure of fund-raising efforts in this social movement.

No one at the conference mentioned the low turnout or its financial implications for the network. However, one important theme running through the conference was the lack of interest in the movement on the part of the clergy and the public. Attendees recognized that whatever interest they had been able to generate had already peaked and was now in decline. Such cycles in attention to an issue are characteristic of social movements, as first pointed out by Anthony Downs (1972) in his now-classic article.

One theme of the conference was the belief that the church had expressed concern about the issue but that it now believed that the problem had been adequately handled and was no longer pressing. Much of the expressed concern, according to those at the conference, did not, however, represent genuine acceptance of the claims by the clergy but was, rather, designed as a public relations effort. They are now smarter about what they say publicly and more expert in damage control. Thus, the problem has been defined as resolved by the church, and SNAP members who do not believe that it is, by any means, over are hard-pressed to reframe it otherwise so that the public and the media remain interested. Much of the discussion at the conference revolved around efforts to interest the media in the issue and a visit to the annual meeting of the Conference Bishops, with whose meeting the SNAP meeting was planned to coincide. Evidence of the church's lack of interest in the issue came from the description by Barbara Blaine, the founder of SNAP, of her efforts to get the bishops to meet with a group of SNAP members. After several efforts to arrange such a meeting, the Bishops' Ad Hoc Committee on Sexual Abuse was willing to see two of the members privately before the bishops' meeting began. For the members of SNAP, who had wanted more bishops to meet more SNAP members, this was a serious disappointment as well as an indication of the lack of responsiveness of the church to their claims.

Despite this rather negative view, the conference leaders strove to keep an upbeat tone. They talked extensively of the importance of personal healing and told many stories of individual activism, however modest. The connection between activism and healing was mentioned specifically. Frank Fitzpatrick of Survivor Connections, who put an ad in the paper that read, "Remember Father Porter," was cited as a positive example. We were told of one member who had the police go to the home of her perpetrator when he was out on parole to require him to register as a sex offender. Another, whose suit failed on statute of limitations grounds, worked on legislation in California to change that law: "I have a voice, I can make a difference." Another threw flyers in the vestibule of the church stating that its priest had abused him. No one really suggested that these gestures had much of an effect on the problem in general; instead, they were considered part of the healing process.

Survivors tell their stories at all conferences. At this one, a significant portion of the conference was devoted to these accounts. The groundwork for this part of the conference was laid very carefully, with one leader stressing several times the importance of confidentiality of what was being said. Several survivors had been selected by the conference leaders, and after they had told their stories, others, inspired by their example, followed them to the microphone. The cathartic effect of this process was obvious; there were a number of scenes of tears and prolonged hugging among the participants. Support was also available from the professional speakers at the conference, one of whom described the participants as "heroes for surviving," while Jeffrey Anderson, a lawyer, opened his talk by saying he was "distinguished by the courage of my clients." At one point, yellow ribbons were passed around, and the participants were encouraged to wear them. For those who needed explanation of this symbol, the analogy that yellow ribbons used to show support of those who fought in the Gulf War was mentioned. "We are heroes, too, though we don't get the recognition. We will be recognized here at least" (Blaine, 1996). This is an adaptation of what Taylor and Whittier (1995) called "feminist practices [which] reinforce new expression rules that dictate open displays of emotion and empathy and legitimate extensive attention to participants' emotions and personal histories" (179). That these "feminist practices" have moved beyond the women's movement is illustrated not only by the SNAP conference but by the displays of hugging at gatherings of traditional men such as the Promise Keepers.

Another interesting feature of the conference was the extent to which it served as a place for survivors to get legal advice about their prospective and current lawsuits. One of the speakers was an attorney, Jeffrey Anderson, who is one of the few experts in clergy abuse cases in the country. He already knew a number of the participants, having represented them in their lawsuits. After he talked about the current state of the law and the response of the church, he held consultations with anyone who wanted to talk to him just outside the conference room while the conference continued. This underwrote one of the themes of the conference expressed by David Clohessy, that lawsuits and media publicity were the two avenues to social change. In addition, it provides further illustration of the development of collective identity for the social movement that uses social institutions to obtain justice and change. The development of a collective identity by the networks is discussed in further detail in the next section.

WHAT NETWORKS DO: DEVELOPING
A COLLECTIVE IDENTITY

Defining What's at Stake

One of the most important roles of networks is the framing work that they do to define the issues on which the social movement is built (Snow and Benford, 1992). As we have seen elsewhere, claims-makers strive for the broadest possible definition of the problem. Survivor Connections, for example, describes its potential members as "people sexually abused by any type of perpetrator, whether the abuse was done to a child or an adult; and for pro-survivors (defined as supportive relatives, friends or significant others of survivors)" (*Survivor Activist* 2.4, 1994: 1). Thus, the frame is extended to the victims of all types of sexual abuse as well as those who have not personally suffered the harm but who are close to someone who has, usually family members or, in the case of the clergy, the congregation. Some conferences have special panels or workshops for these pro-survivors (e.g., To Tell the Truth, 1994). The frame is further enhanced by those who declare that anyone can be a victim of professional sexual misconduct. This serves the purpose of stressing the "normality" of the victims as well as their ubiquity. At one conference, the phrase "we are all abusers" was constantly repeated to reinforce this framework (Restoring the Integrity Conference, 1993). Thus, all the audience becomes involved in the development of a collective identity, including those who have not personally been victimized.

At conferences and in newsletters, the frame is amplified, its causes clarified appropriately, and certain solutions advocated and others rejected. Certain appropriate terms and phrases are used frequently, such as "breach of trust," "empowerment," "abuse of power," "boundary violation," "vulnerability," and "the power of healing." Victims are described as "survivors," "triumphant survivors," "heroes," "courageous for the act of surviving and coming forward." All these terms both frame the problem in a particular way and also encourage participants' positive feelings about themselves and the group to which they belong.

Evidence of the widespread existence of the problem is an important element of framing. For example, Survivor Connections' newsletter, called the *Survivor Activist*, routinely lists descriptions of cases of interest both in the United States and around the world. These are often cases in which members of the clergy have been charged or convicted on sexual abuse or pedophilia charges. *Missing Link* has a similar section that it calls "Black Collar Crimes."[6] We learn, for example, of such small details as the plea-bargaining negotiations by Father Gordon MacRae in the Superior Court in Keene, New Hampshire (*Survivor Activist* 3.1, 1995). He was subsequently convicted and received a "much more just sentence" of 33 years (8). We also learn that in Catlettsburg, Kentucky, Rev. William Blankenship, "acquitted last fall of sodomizing a 12-year-old boy, was convicted of sodomizing another boy, 14" (*Missing Link* 3.2, 1995: 9). The implication here, of course, is that Rev. Blankenship was guilty of both charges, though the legal system was unable to convict him on the first one. These case descriptions can be seen as efforts to alter the traditional cultural codings in our society (Swidler, 1986). Traditionally, the clergy, in particular, are viewed as better than us mere mortals, perhaps a bit more than human, and certainly unselfish and beneficent. In the context of this social movement they are being presented as criminals who are mean, base, and selfish. This is part of a general willingness to question members of the clergy described by Philip Jenkins (1996). The "Black Collar Crimes" section of *Missing Link* includes not just sexual crimes but all crimes by the clergy. Unlike the myth of the Catholic priest as above earthly sexual desires, these priests are not only sexual but also willing to take advantage of their positions of power and the high public esteem in which they are held. By the same token, the traditional views of the church as being unselfishly interested in the welfare of its adherents is also altered by publicity indicating that the church is unwilling to take responsibility for the abuse of its representatives, which is exhibited in the strong defense mounted in many recent cases of clergy sexual abuse.

Newsletters and meetings provide information about legislation that is part of the framing of the issue. For example, Survivor Connections reports on the fate of "Megan's law," the law requiring that the public be notified when a convicted sex offender is released from prison. Frequent mention is made at clergy abuse conferences on developments in statutes of limitations, which is a central issue in many of the civil cases pursued by victims.

Sexual abuse as a worldwide problem is emphasized by the networks. The 1997 Linkup Conference was advertised through the slogan "Clergy Sexual Abuse: A Global Crisis." Newsletters use examples from abroad in support of the international nature of the problem. For example, *Survivor Connections* informs us that in Saudi Arabia the usual punishment for rape is death. "This year several perpetrators have been beheaded," *Survivor Activist* reports with apparent approval (3.2, 1995: 8). In England a rapist who has randomly attacked 13 women is now a suspect in four more rapes in East Leeds, while in Italy Chinese children are said to have been sold for sex (*Survivor Activist* 3.2, 1995: 7; 5.2, 1997: 9). In Dublin Father Brendan Smyth died shortly after beginning to serve a 12-year sentence after pleading guilty to 74 instances of the sexual abuse of 20 young people over a period of 36 years (*Missing Link*, 1997: 15). Both Western and non-Western countries are cited in a variety of contexts to reinforce the breadth of the problem. In one newsletter, the number of survivors is given as 750 million around the world (*Proclamations of Survivor Connections*, n.d.), and the "dream" of these .75 billion survivors in a global march is mentioned in another newsletter (*Survivor Activist*, 1998: 2) In general, there is a rather tabloid quality to these reports, with emphasis on the horror story as activating agent. Statistics are also used to shock and are framed in stark and simple terms. If different studies provide varying incidence rates, the highest will be the most attractive for citation at conferences and in newsletters. Accuracy does not seem to be as important as big numbers; the figures given in *The Survivor Activist* are said to total over 3,300, but simple addition brings the number to 2,944. It is often difficult to obtain information about the nature of the research used to develop these data or even their source. Networks are not interested in reporting academic research but rather in presenting "information" in support of the international and extensive nature of sexual abuse as a means of developing collective solidarity and to channel emotions of outrage and identification with other sufferers (Taylor and Whittier, 1995).

Telling Members What to Think: The Development of Group Norms

The newsletters and the conferences play an important role in the development and continuity of group norms and identity. They are very outspoken in their views of the issues involved. The enemy is clearly defined as "perps," for whom the most serious punishment is appropriate, as well as the church, which must be "called to account."

Belief in the existence of repressed memory and ritual abuse is a central norm, and those who discredit repressed memory, especially the False Memory Syndrome Foundation, are also depicted as the enemy. To counter the claims of those who argue that memories in these cases can be false (as in "false memory syndrome"), networks call it "true memory syndrome," and Survivor Connections uses the logo "The True Memory Foundation" in the masthead to their introductory package. Survivor Connections denies that repressed memory could ever be inaccurate, while the more moderate *Missing Link* states, "Without judging the merits of any single case, society needs to acknowledge . . . the reality of repressed memory" (*Missing Link* 3.1, 1995). The 1997 Linkup Conference devoted extensive attention to describing the nature of the defense based on false memory, especially in court.

Network response to the revelation that Steven Cook acknowledged that his charges against Cardinal Bernardin were false illustrates this well (*Survivor Activist* 2.4, 1994). The newsletter criticized Cook's acknowledgment that his "memories" were obtained under hypnosis as a "ploy . . . that his therapist is somehow to blame. In reality, Steven Cook should take full personal responsibility for his own actions" (1). The danger of "blaming" the therapist is clearly that it might serve to discredit other therapists who play a central role in the movement to recover memories of sexual abuse. Another network newsletter described in some detail the "healing of Steven Cook and Cardinal Bernardin, who participated in a "very moving and profound healing moment in both their lives" (*Missing Link*, 3.1, 1995: 3). What the description neglects to mention is that the "simple and direct" apologies were by Cook, who admitted that his charges against Bernardin were false[7] (Niebuhr, 1994). This issue was addressed by one of the speakers at the Linkup conference who described Cook as saying that he "needed to believe that Bernardin didn't do it" after the meeting he had with the cardinal (Whitfield, 1997). This, combined with the assertion that Cook did not retract his accusation of abuse by the other priest, left the field muddied, to say the least.

Despite the response of the networks, this case is clearly a roadblock in the movement, as illustrated by the attorney Jeffrey Anderson, who said at the SNAP conference (November 1996) that the Catholic Church has become "more brazen" in litigating cases, in part because of that case. It represents the dominant cultural view that people who claim to have repressed memories of sexual abuse are making them up and are therefore not to be taken seriously by the church or the public. Anderson presents the more moderate of the claims-makers' view, buttressed by his personal experience as a plaintiff's attorney in these cases, that false memory is "so rare it is tantamount to nonexistent."

Positions taken at the more academic conferences are generally less overt but nevertheless strong. Books written by those whose views match their own are recommended, while those whose views differ are criticized. The book exhibits at conferences are a veritable catalog of the norms of the movement, with no representation from those whose views are mixed or different from the received wisdom.

The networks also provide ongoing commentary on well-known cases. The best example of this is the Father Porter case, mentioned before as the reason for the founding of Survivor Connections. Father Porter was alleged to have molested over 100 children over a period of years in a variety of parishes, resulting in many civil and criminal suits filed against him (Butterfield, 1992a; "Ex-Priest Gets Jail," 1993). The networks' interest in this case is particularly strong for several reasons. First, it supports one of their claims, which is that members of the clergy who engage in sexual abuse of their parishioners have been moved away from the location of these activities to another location, where the behavior continues. It also provides evidence of the claim that this is a huge problem simply by virtue of the number of victims who have come forward. The networks claim that many other victims have not come forward, despite encouragement by them to do so. Cases such as Father Porter's can be used to support the assertion in a newsletter that "[statistics] show that most perpetrators do not get caught until after 200 victims" (*Survivor Connections Introductory Package*, n.d.: 5). This case is also, as mentioned before, a matter of personal importance to the movement because Frank Fitzpatrick, the founder of Survivor Connections, was himself abused by Father Porter. Much of his activism has revolved around his efforts to bring Porter to justice, and the network was begun out of that activism; it is clearly a flagship case in the movement. It exemplifies the "enemy" for the movement: one who abused vast numbers of people and got away with it because the victims were reluctant to come forward and also because he was protected by his institution. Frequent referral to Father Porter provides a focus for the revulsion that is essential for the collective solidarity of a diverse group. The flame is fanned regularly in the newsletters; the Spring 1998 issue of *Survivor Activist* includes a calculation of the number of days remaining until Father Porter is eligible for parole (under the heading "Vulture Alert").

Much has been made by the organizations of the $120 million verdict in a case against several priests and the diocese of Dallas. This case is a major victory for the movement, as it provides legal recognition of the claims that the church has been engaged in a cover-up of both the problem of clergy sexual abuse and the way it has handled it. *Missing Link*, in describing the case, says that it "not only ignited an international media frenzy, but has dealt the Roman Catholic Church a huge blow, denting their once-believed indestructible armor" (1997: 1). The 1997 Linkup conference devoted an entire evening to the case, with a tape of *Larry King Live* and a presentation by the attorney for several of the plaintiffs. The case provided a source of solidarity and vindication of their cause as well as a clear illustration of a successful outcome for those who take on the church in civil court.

The results of civil suits are not always so positive, and the newsletters take pains to address those issues as well. When the Supreme Court of California refused to hear the arguments of plaintiffs suing the diocese in the case involving Father Ted Llanos, it was reported in detail by Tom Economous, president of the Linkup, in the newsletter *Missing Link* (Economous, 1999). Economous used the opportunity to challenge the cardinal of the Los Angeles diocese to "step up to assist these men" rather than continuing to deny that the church is responsible and spending time raising "40 million dollars for a new cathedral that no one wants or needs" (Economous, 1999: 1). This focuses readers' attention on the need for a realignment of the priorities of the church so the claims of abused victims can be addressed.

Positions are taken on other issues that serve both to identify norms and to provide a basis for individual and collective action. Megan's law, mentioned earlier, is strongly supported by the networks. The spring 1998 issue of *The Survivor Activist* contains detailed suggestions for ways to encourage more states to join the national sex offender registry, including model letters to write to various public officials. Networks also support long sentences for perpetrators, as, for example, when a newsletter reports that a jury in Oklahoma recommended a 30,000-year sentence for a man convicted of raping a three-year-old girl (*Survivor Activist* 3.1, 1995: 1). They disapprove strongly of gag orders, which civil litigants are often asked to sign, requiring silence by the plaintiff about settlement of the lawsuit. One newsletter devoted extensive attention to gag orders and to ways of circumventing or defying them (*Survivor Activist* 3.1, 1995: 4–6). At the 1997 Linkup conference, several questions on the issue were addressed to lawyers with expertise on the issue. As we have seen in connection with the recovered memory debate, statutes of limitations are also disapproved of because they are central to the viability of many claims and can prevent victims from filing for civil remedies on the basis of events that occurred years ago. Newsletters and conferences devote time to the current state of the law on this issue and suggest legislative changes as a focus for activism among members (Linkup Conference, 1997; SNAP conference, 1996; *Survivor Activist* 2.2, 1994: 7).

The networks are also concerned that they take "ownership" of the problem. In one newsletter, Tom Economous describes the need to reclaim the survivors movement, which, he argues, has lost the power to control itself (*Missing Link* 3.2, 1995: 1). The "cause, or purpose, and in this case, the victims have been eclipsed" by journalists, authors, attorneys, and academic forums and those who have "garnered fame and fortune from our molestation" and "the vultures who feed on this social problem," "high-profile attorneys who have made a career out of our pain." This sentiment is echoed by one of the founders of the Forbidden Zone self-help group when describing the group's plans to organize a conference: "[W]e are going to ask Rutter, Gartrell, and John Weiner" (all professionals who specialize in various aspects of the problem). "We want to be the authorities and have these people just come and speak briefly" (Parker, 1997). This effort to be the official representative of the problem works two ways. On one hand, it provides group members with the solidarity of exclusivity, while, on the other, it works against mobilization by excluding from participation in the movement those who have not suffered personally. This need to "own" the problem stands in contrast to the expansionist view expressed earlier, exemplified by the slogans "anyone can be a victim" and "we are all offenders." On one hand, the movement wants to be inclusive; on the other, it wants to limit membership to those who have personally suffered. This ambivalence may be connected to the fear that outsiders, like lawyers and journalists, are part of the problem rather than the solution and may, in part, explain why relatively few people not directly affected by professional sexual misconduct join the networks.

In addition to these explicit positions taken by the networks, implicit norms guide the activities of groups. At more academic conferences, the norms may not be as openly expressed as they are elsewhere in the movement. Nevertheless, when someone presents a session about professional sexual exploitation entitled "Misconduct or Misunderstanding," it is clear that we are to understand that the behavior is misconduct rather than misunderstanding. The titles of conferences themselves have strong normative and political overtones. For example, one conference was called Restoring the Integrity: An Educational Conference on the Dimensions of Sexual Exploitation by Professions Involved in Relationships of Trust. The implication is that professionals have lost integrity and that the conference is designed to alter that situation. Calling the Church to Account, the title of the 1997 Linkup conference, implies that the church has something to account for. By the same token, a conference called To Tell the Truth implies that previous information has been false, while one called From Surviving to Thriving provides a positive statement about individual healing. None of these gatherings have much place for anyone who disagrees with the views expressed; instead of challenging questions from the audience, there is a sea of earnest nodding in response to the speakers.

Providing Support and Information

Like the support groups, the networks serve an important role in offering emotional support and listening on an individual basis to the narratives of those who have been victimized. They, too, have telephone lines, staffed by survivors, available both for those who wish to remain anonymous and those who are willing to give their names. One of the slogans of Survivor Connections is that "you are no longer alone," which is borne out in the use of the telephone hot line as well as the other services offered by the networks. Support is also available through a fairly active correspondence on relevant issues among the subscribers to the newsletter. One correspondent wrote: "I could not believe the perfect timing of the summer 1994 *Survivor Activist* newsletter! The article entitled 'More Victims: The Price of Silence,' and the information it contained was exactly what I have been agonizing about for the past two weeks." The correspondent goes on to tell her story and asks such questions as to how "can we address this issue? How can we advocate for others?" (*Survivor Activist* 2.4, 1994: 3).

This support and the development of group narratives through the hearing of stories are also a central part of the conferences. At every conference, time is set aside for volunteers to tell their stories to the group as a way of constructing shared meanings. In each case, issues of confidentiality are discussed at length, as a way both to protect the individual storyteller and also to stress that breach of confidentiality is one of the "violations" members have suffered as part of their shared past experience. Thus, this violation becomes part of the shared cultural understanding of what defines the movement. However, the reluctance of many members to tell their stories outside the meeting reduces their effectiveness as a mobilizing tool. Only when someone "goes public" to the media can the general public gain an understanding of the nature of the problem, and can other sufferers define themselves as potential members of the movement and actually participate in movement activities.

Conferences provide another kind of support, both for survivors and for those who work with them. They provide the sense that there are others out there in the same position. The isolation of victims of professional sexual misconduct has been documented elsewhere in this book, but the professionals, the lawyers and therapists who work in this "obscure" area, also feel a sense of isolation and even disapproval from colleagues. As one lawyer put it at a conference: "[I]t's a breath of fresh air to talk without being challenged (Roseman, 1998).

The emotional support provided by the organizations is very broad and extends even to offering condolences to members for the loss of loved ones. Members are made to feel that others take a personal interest even in those aspects of their lives that do not relate to the victimization itself. Such is the feeling of group solidarity that the term "family" is used frequently.

The newsletters are also a forum for the dissemination of information about events that might be of interest to the subscribers, such as conferences, workshops, and retreats. One newsletter has a regular column for people looking for information about alleged sexual abusers (*Missing Link*). They are also used for the solicitation of research subjects by professionals undertaking research in this field. The organization Stop It Now, for example, which "is continuing its research into the characteristics of sexual abuse perpetrators," offers to send its confidential questionnaire to willing respondents (*Survivor Activist* 2.4, 1994: 12). One university-affiliated research project placed an insert in a newsletter looking for women and men of color who have been exploited by a variety of professional care providers, while a psychologist-priest had a sign-up sheet at the 1997 Linkup conference. It is unclear whether these researchers have been checked out by the organizers, but it is clear that the way they frame the problem is more important than their credentials as scientific researchers.

For newcomers to the movement, conferences and network newsletters provide more academic information about the framework of the problem through the sale of recommended books or tapes on the subject, including taped transcripts of its most recent conference (Missing Link; It's Never O.K.). Information about the nature and the scope of the problem is also usually presented at the conferences, though the ones that are survivor-controlled devote little attention to it, perhaps because they assume that their audience has already developed an identity based on group norms that include recognition of the serious nature of the problem. At academic conferences, much of the information is already published, but it is presented in an audience-friendly way. It is also combined with more personal insights and sometimes the narrative of the presenter's own experience, which serves to liven up the empirical material and give the presenter credibility as a member of the group.

Get Out There and Do Something: Mobilization

As resource mobilization theory makes clear, social movement organizations play a central role in mobilizing members to take collective action (Jenkins, 1983). Newsletters and conferences provide what Snow and Benford (1988) describe as the call to arms. Here is the place where people are motivated to do something about professional sexual exploitation and are given the rationale for that action. At conferences, the members of the audience are seen as both potential activists themselves and as a conduit to others. One speaker said: "[I]f you are not part of the solution, you're part of the problem" (Marshall, 1998). At one such conference in Houston, the brochure used a quote from Elie Wiesel: "Let us remember: What hurts the victim most is not the cruelty of the oppressor but the silence of the bystander." The closing remarks echoed this theme by telling the audience that they had "broken the silence pact of the past today, and there are no bystanders in this room."[8] The idea that the silence surrounding the problem is some kind of conspiracy is a central norm of the professional sexual misconduct movement that is used in several ways; here it is a rallying cry for action.

There is usually a designedly optimistic quality to this aspect of the conferences. Rather than becoming depressed by the information about the terrible problem, the audience is encouraged to turn this knowledge into something positive by engaging in activism. Even at the SNAP conference, the least upbeat of the conferences, considerable time was devoted to stories of individuals who took action that they defined as successful, a "happy ending" that showed that victory was possible for others also. The actions had a David and Goliath quality about them and usually involved one person against the parish, the school board, or the church itself. The expressed message was that one individual can make a difference, a classic mobilization cry that in this case is meant literally, rather than with the implication that the one person would get together with others.

In a few cases, the nature of the activism is actually specified. The letter-writing campaign to extend "Megan's law" in *The Survivor Activist* was discussed earlier. The Houston Conference resulted in the formation of the Houston Coalition on Sexual Misconduct, which subsequently played a role in lobbying for the passage of legislation providing civil and criminal penalties for professional sexual misconduct in Texas (Alexander, 1993a). Efforts to negotiate a meeting with the bishops described earlier in the SNAP case study are another specific example. At the same SNAP conference and also at the Linkup conference, the organizers circulated a how-to document written for a different purpose, to show members how to work toward passing appropriate statutes with the recommendation that activists try to extend the statute of limitations in their states. The latest effort, outlined at the 1997 Linkup conference, addresses third-party liability, which is covered by the usual period of limitation and therefore provides a barrier to suits against the church.

For the most part, the actions suggested are rather general and usually not organized by the group; rather, it is expected that individual members will take them on, either alone or with the help of others whom they enlist. There is little attempt to organize protests or marches as is so common in other social movements. Suggestions for group activities are usually for the benefit of individuals rather than for the cause itself and belong more in the category of support group activity than collective action. The networks do not appear to care much whether the actions are identified as coming from their members (Clohessy, 1995).

Networks, like self-help groups, are geared more toward the provision of information about how to take individual, rather than collective, action. As we have seen, *The Survivor Activist* is the most direct of the newsletters in its advice. For the most part, however, as we have seen in the case study earlier, it is avowedly uninterested in collective action. Rather, it offers suggestions, for example, on how to deal with the requests of lawyers for the defense for gag orders or suggestions for violating them once having signed them. It also suggests ways in which a victim can confront his or her "perp," even including a "dead perp." Such suggestions range from telling as many people as possible about the events, to taping one's perpetrator, to conducting a ceremony in front of friends and supporters, to a mock trial (*Survivor Activist* 3.2, 1995: 1–3). Clearly, these latter suggestions do not serve to punish the perpetrators but are instead intended to help the survivors in their recovery process. All these suggestions are framed in ways that attempt to realign the power balance between the individual and the institution perceived to be the source of the problem. The network is anxious to make clear that it, rather than the church, holds the moral high ground, which puts potential illegal behavior, like violating a gag order or taping someone's conversation without permission, into the category of civil disobedience rather than lawbreaking.

Using the Media in Framing the Issue

As with all social movements, connection to the media is a constant issue with networks and conferences. They seek to provide the media with a neatly packaged representation of the problem. Newsletters frequently list the talk shows on which a particular leader has made an appearance, as do the biographies in conference announcements. The more academic conferences provide a focus for transmitting serious information about the social problem to the media, though this is often not picked up because of the greater attraction of the talk-show approach. As Tarrow (1994) and others have pointed out, the media are themselves involved in the framing process, and members of the organizations often express frustration at their inability to control the media. This may be because they feel that their framework is not being accurately presented by the media or, worse, that they are being ignored. At the Fredericton Conference, concern was expressed about "tabloid journalism" (i.e., inappropriately framing the problem), and access to the conference by the media was limited. More commonly, the media are invited and do not attend, as was the case at the SNAP conference, thus diminishing the publicity and the importance of the problem in the eyes of members. The ambivalence was obvious at the 1997 Linkup conference, where Brooks Edgerton, a journalist for the *Dallas Morning News*, who has done considerable investigative reporting about the case against the diocese of Dallas as well as related issues, was lauded for his work by one speaker and told to leave the session by another.

SO HOW WELL DO THEY WORK? MEASURES OF "SUCCESS" AND "FAILURE"

How well these organizations succeed or fail in their various goals is, as we have already seen, a complex question of interpretation and perception. It is also a question that can be addressed to the whole movement or to parts of it, like a conference or a response by a group targeted for activism. With respect to the networks and the meetings, there are some objective measures to consider.

The size and number of organizations are obvious indicators of the size (and importance) of a movement. By that measure, professional sexual exploitation is a very small and insignificant problem. As far as can be determined, total membership of the three main networks numbers about 13,000, including overlap. Of those, the lion's share are survivors themselves, with virtually all the rest of the membership limited to family members and those whose professional interests involve them in the issue, like lawyers and therapists, rather than those who have a general concern about the issue. For those who discover the existence of a network, the experience can be a salutary one; the network does provide them with a way of defining what happened to them or to someone near to them. It provides a focus for future behavior, in terms of both personal healing and individual and group action. But these networks, unlike those in other organizations, do not provide an ongoing cadre of activists. Once the network has served its healing and informational purpose, for most individuals the incentive to belong diminishes considerably. That is no doubt why the networks are so involved in trying to get their members to pay their dues in an effort to stem the tide of membership turnover. One network had a membership drive contest to encourage new membership, offering as prizes such benefits as free air fare to the next Linkup conference and lifelong membership in the organization (*Missing Link* 2.2, 1994: 2). The problem of loss of members is also why it is so easy for the networks to go through periods of being moribund or even to collapse altogether.

The perennial lack of money troubles all organizations devoted to social change. Here, however, it is bad enough to curtail the activities of the networks and make it impossible for them to hire any paid help. This reliance on volunteers is also, of course, typical of all social movements, but here again it is bad enough to contribute to burnout by leaders, who are often not replaced by someone equally dedicated. Unlike other organizations, none of these networks receive much outside funding, either from the government or private sources, with the small exception of money for scholarships to go to conferences. Like the self-help groups, funding issues have political significance; the Linkup takes money from the church, whereas the other networks do not (Clohessy, 1995). The Linkup is also the only group that has any paid help; its president, Tom Economous, works full-time for the organization, which is also the most successful.

In the case of conferences, one basic indicator of success or lack thereof is whether a planned conference actually takes place. As we saw in the case of support groups, the history of conferences in the area of professional sexual misconduct has by no means been all smooth sailing. There have been conferences that have been successful, for example, the It's Never O.K. conference described earlier and the Boston and Sydney conferences, as well as the Linkup conferences for survivors. After the It's Never O.K. conference, the momentum seemed to diminish, but subsequent conferences have been eventually held. Because there is no stable organization to take control on a regular basis, there is always the question of who will take the initiative to organize the next meeting. More than one conference has been planned but has not taken place. As Gary Schoener put it at the 1998 Boston conference, "[E]very time we have one of these things, I worry about it going on again." Survivor Connections seems to be suffering from the same loss of momentum; the autumn 1996 newsletter says: "This year we decided not to put on a conference since we did not have time or energy to do it right, perhaps sometime next year we will be able to plan one" (*Survivor Activist* 1996: 1). Now they see their role as coordinating the efforts of the regional groups who put on To Tell the Truth conferences.

Another measure of success is the number of people who actually attend meetings. Interpretation of the attendance is, of course, somewhat self-fulfilling; if one plans for only a small audience, and the enrollment exceeds expectations, the organizers can label the conference a success. About 300–400 participants seem to be the norm of the successful conferences, often helped by the central and attractive location in which they are held (Boston, Sydney, Toronto). At the other extreme, however, numbers below a certain minimum are a clear indicator of failure and can result in cancellation, as happened with the attempt to hold an It's Never O.K. conference in 1988. In the case of the SNAP conference, it took place despite having only about 30 attendees, but such small numbers meant it did not raise the much-needed funds as the organizers apparently hoped it would. Failure, either through cancellation or an embarrassingly small audience, does the movement untold harm. It shows to anyone who learns about it that the social problem is not really serious and leads to a loss of morale and defection of members.

Another indicator of success or failure is whether the call to activism in the newsletters and conferences produces results. In a few cases there is evidence that it does. As mentioned earlier, the Houston conference resulted directly in the setting up of a task force and indirectly in the passage of legislation. After attending an early It's Never O.K. conference in Minneapolis, Theresa Donahue, who was involved in the sunrise/sunset provisions of professional regulation statutes in Colorado in 1988, decided to include criminal provisions against professional sexual misconduct in the revised statute. By contrast, members of SNAP failed in their efforts to have a major meeting with the bishops during their Washington conference, which meant no action by the bishops and, perhaps more importantly, no media publicity of their conference or their cause. There have, however, been no major organized initiatives resulting from conferences.

Increased membership in a network is also a measure of success, as was the case after several Survivor Connections conferences. The opposite can

also be true. After the failure of the organizers to set up the 1988 conference, an organization responsible for setting up the conference, the
Association against Sex in Client Therapy, "had their back broken by the
failure of the conference and went under" (Schoener, 24 June 1993).

A further measure of success is the extent and variety of the cosponsorship of a conference or network. This is both an illustration of links to
other organizations and movements and an indication of the effectiveness
of the movement itself. It also contributes to the success of a conference by
providing seed money for initial publicity, as well as providing a ready-
made target audience for that publicity. The more academic conferences
are more likely to have such cosponsorship, though even survivor conferences are also cosponsored for reasons of finance rather than respectability. The To Tell the Truth conferences put on by Survivor Connections have
been cosponsored by student groups at the university where they were
held and by a law firm.

Media interest is much harder to measure as an indicator of success or
failure of the organizations and their activities. There is some evidence
from interviews with those deeply involved in the subject that it is increasingly difficult to catch the attention of the media to report on the organizations, illustrating the "down" of the issue attention cycle (Schoener,
21 October 1996; Blaine, 1996; Downs, 1972). Certain newsworthy events
can trigger renewed interest, as happened in the case of the Dallas verdict,
but there seems to be less momentum for future reporting generated by
that interest.

CONCLUSION

To the extent that social movement success can be defined as organized
efforts to precipitate social change that leads to tangible results, this movement falls far short. As we have seen, the organizations rarely mobilize
their members into organized protest or other group activity. Frank
Fitzpatrick, for example, the founder of Survivor Connections, specifically
expressed his lack of interest in collective action. In this social movement
any organized activity is undertaken by members on their own, and, while
it is applauded by other members and their leaders, it is not seen as an essential requirement of membership in the movement. Many in the movement see it in both personal and collective terms, and to the extent that
individual and group goals conflict, they opt for emphasis on individual
goals. Because they have so few members who are not involved in personal healing from the effects of professional sexual misconduct, there is
no base from which to draw activists not currently involved in personal recovery. Because the organizations did not emerge from other organizations or institutions, they have nowhere to look for members and support.
Those few people who are active are seen as having already "done their

healing." However, most people who have done their healing drop out of the movement. Thus, these networks and conferences are not very successful in mobilizing and undertaking collective action. As we have seen, however, the networks and the conferences do serve their members well in providing the tools for their recovery from professional sexual exploitation. They provide information, support, and a collective identity. Thus, if success is defined as the achievement of *both* individual and group goals, the networks and conferences can readily be classified as successful. Such an approach brings us back to the view that framing is everything, including the definition of success and failure.

NOTES

1. For an extended list of related organizations, see *The Survivor Activist* 6.1 (Spring 1998), and the Web site http://www.advocateweb.com.

2. In fact, the numbers they give add up to 2,944, of whom 1,487 are professionals, and the others fit a variety of categories, including survivors of incest, rape, and ritual abuse.

3. Many of the victims I have spoken to have been obtained through my placing an announcement on the Web site.

4. The numbering system is rather strange, as the 1996 conference in Sydney, Australia, was billed as the fourth in a series on this theme, while the 1998 Boston Conference was also called the fourth international conference.

5. By that description, about the only person present who had no expertise was the author, whose status as part of the movement has been questioned more than once!

6. *The Missing Link* also includes a section on crimes against the clergy, further evidence that it is more balanced than the newsletter of Survivor Connections.

7. Cardinal Bernardin, in a book published posthumously, made an allegation that a priest encouraged Cook to charge Bernardin with sexual abuse, an allegation that the priest denies ("Priest Denies Targeting Cardinal," 1997).

8. The Houston Conference on Sexual Misconduct by Clergy, Psychotherapists and Health Care Professionals, Houston, Texas, 26 February 1993. Remarks presented by Joan Alexander, Conference Chair.

— 6 —

THE LAW

This is the "age of litigation." The potential exposure to the Catholic Church for the continuation of claimants coming forward . . . is very great. . . . It might have been unthinkable a few years ago for a Catholic parent to sue the Church. Similarly, there was a time when it was un-thinkable for a patient to sue a physician.

—Peterson, 1985

INTRODUCTION

In the Anglo-American legal system, new law develops in patchwork fash-ion to fill perceived gaps and in response to changing social attitudes. The gaps may become visible through publicity about "new" social wrongs for which there is apparently no legal remedy. Claims are frequently but-tressed by social science research documenting the seriousness of the problem. In developing new case law, practicing lawyers take cases in ar-eas when they consider the law ripe for change; scholars write articles sug-gesting the application of legal doctrine previously used in analogous areas; judges accept the more expansive arguments in cases before them. At the same time, legislators may take steps to fill the gaps by passing leg-islation aimed at the social problem. In the course of all this activity, the actors work to frame or reframe the problem in ways that are most con-ducive to legal remedies. In response to this activity, other players, includ-ing defendants, courts, and insurers, may use various techniques to resist this expansion.

So it is with professional sexual misconduct. As we have seen, the issue has been brought to public attention over the last couple of decades. De-velopments in case law and legislation have followed the pattern just described. Case law has been developed because lawyers who were previously not willing to take such cases now do so, based, in part, on the public interest and the incidence research, as well as publicity about successful cases. There have been a few articles on the subject, though hardly a flood, and not until 1995 was a text published on the subject (Bisbing et al., 1995). Those publications have, however, provided the groundwork for the inclusion of professional sexual misconduct into current law and the application of nontraditional legal doctrines to it. The text by Bisbing et al. provides a particularly instructive model of the legal refocusing and reframing process in professional sexual misconduct. It is a combination of a description of current law laced with suggestions of strategies to be used by attorneys to reframe and expand legal claims.

It has long been an article of faith in the United States that the law is a powerful instrument for social change. Some scholars have argued, however, that, instead, it serves a diversionary purpose by focusing people's attention on legal activities like lawsuits and legislative change, rather than on other activities that might better serve the goals of social movement activists. In the case of professional sexual misconduct, the focus is on the law, almost to the exclusion of other activity. Legal mechanisms are used for the financial and psychological benefit of the individual plaintiff, a goal that is highly approved by social movement activists. The underlying hope is that individual judgments or, more often, settlements will somehow bring about social change. Success through the legal system can be evaluated both in individual terms (did the plaintiff win?) and in social terms (have lawsuits and legislative developments had a beneficial effect on the nature and extent of the social problem?).

Much of this legal analysis has taken place in an atheoretical environment. Recent developments in feminist legal theory provide an instructive framework within which to evaluate changes in the law of professional sexual misconduct. The extensive recent scholarship in feminist legal theory is beyond the scope of this book. For the purposes of this book, however, feminist legal theory can illustrate the ways in which the law exists within the gendered framework of a patriarchal legal system. Some feminist legal scholars have applied the theory to substantive areas of the law, with particular emphasis on those acts of violence in which women are primarily the victims (e.g., rape and domestic violence). Others have shown the various ways in which tort law and especially recent reforms in tort law have worked to the disadvantage of women (Bender, 1993; Koenig and Rustad 1995). Koenig and Rustad (1995), for example, show that punitive damages are often awarded in sexual misconduct cases; not surprisingly, the plaintiffs are usually female. These punitive damages are seriously affected by recent tort reforms that provide for "caps" (financial upper limits) on the amounts awarded (64).

The central claim of "difference feminism," as the most recent theoretical approach is called, is that "the legal subjecthood to which women had been assimilated was implicitly male, and that possibly the very methods of legal practices were masculine" (Lacey, 1998: 192). Thus, cases of violence against women are handled in the legal system using a model of male behavior and male methods. The male is the norm against which all behavior is measured. Perceptions of reasonable behavior and beliefs are also male.

The aim of the rest of this chapter is twofold. First, it describes the several components of the framing and reframing of professional sexual misconduct within the law.[1] Second, it shows the ways in which legal developments in professional sexual exploitation continue to take place within the patriarchal model described by feminist legal theorists.

APPLICATION OF BASIC LEGAL DOCTRINE

For the most common type of professional sexual exploitation, which is by psychotherapists, a legal remedy already existed, although it had not been applied to this behavior. As we have seen, in the 1970s there was some question about whether patients' sexual encounters with therapists were harmful; professional opinion has long since changed into a very clear understanding that sexual activity between therapist and patient is always wrong. It is now a clear violation of policies published by the various professional associations. Accordingly, the law that is applied to other forms of medical malpractice applies equally to sexual exploitation by therapists. As early as 1975, in *Roy v. Hartogs*, the plaintiff was able to prove that the sexual relationship she had with her therapist fitted the legal requirements of malpractice. Dr. Hartogs convinced Ms. Roy that a sexual relationship was a necessary part of her treatment. The court held that the therapist's behavior was a breach of the fiduciary duty he owed his patient.[2]

Victims of professional sexual exploitation can sue on the basis of either the professional's negligence or an intentional tort. To succeed in a claim based on negligence, a plaintiff must show (1) that some duty or obligation exists, recognized by the law, that the defendant conform to a certain standard of conduct; (2) that there was a breach of this duty; (3) that there is a reasonable causal link between the behavior complained of and the damage suffered by the plaintiff; and (4) that the plaintiff suffered real damage. In standard cases of professional sexual misconduct, these elements of negligence are not difficult to prove. For example, a therapist certainly owes a duty of care toward his patient, and having a sexual relationship with her is clearly a breach of that duty. It is also fairly easy to prove that the plaintiff was harmed and that harm was caused by the exploitation. A fiduciary is someone who is supposed to behave for the benefit of the person for whom one is acting in that capacity (like a trustee or the guardian of a child). The claim of a breach of fiduciary duty, as in the case of *Roy v. Hartogs*, makes proof easier, as the law generally acknowledges that a fiduciary (in this case the professional) is held to a higher standard of care than an ordinary person. The patriarchal legal system emphasizes the need to guard the safety of those perceived as in need of male protection, in this case, vulnerable women.

Problems may arise when the defendant argues that the sexual exploitation of which the plaintiff complains never took place. This defense can be connected to a description of the plaintiff as someone who would fabricate a sexual relationship as part of her disorder. Such a defense, used frequently in these cases, is a particular twist to the belief, common in rape cases, of a woman as a liar, bent on destroying the reputation of an innocent male. In rape cases the rules of evidence continue to stress the greater than usual likelihood that the complainant is lying, because "women are only too eager to lie about what men have or have not done to them" (Tong, 1984: 100–101). Added to the usual perception of woman as liar is the additional belief of woman as unstable and emotional, nicely buttressed by the fact that the plaintiff sought therapy. A current popular version of woman as liar may stem from what is known as the false memory syndrome, in which memories of earlier sexual abuse recovered in therapy are found to be false.

APPLICATION OF EXISTING DOCTRINE TO NEW DEFENDANTS AND NEW SITUATIONS

A plaintiff may prefer, for reasons of insurance, strategy, or the deeper pockets available for damages, to sue the employer or supervisor of the professional who exploited her.[3] She can use either the doctrine of *respondeat superior* (also known as vicarious liability) or negligent hiring, supervision, or retention. In the case of suits against employers, courts have ruled both for and against plaintiffs, with some courts resisting an expansion of the claim, on the basis that sexual misconduct is not part of the employee's professional services and therefore not the responsibility of the employer (Bisbing et al., 1995: 192–95). In their efforts to push those courts that are reluctant to allow this expansion of liability, Bisbing et al. suggest that lawyers can use a "degree of creativity often precluded in other, more settled, areas of the law" (199).

Suing Third Parties

"Respondeat Superior" or Vicarious Liability

For the plaintiff to succeed in a claim of vicarious liability for professional sexual exploitation, the therapist has to be an employee of the agency and not an independent contractor. In the case of clergy sexual misconduct, the church has argued that priests are independent contractors rather than employees, and therefore the church owes no duty to protect parishioners.

A plaintiff must also prove that the conduct was within the scope of the employment. The plaintiff must confront the argument by the third party that sex cannot be considered to be within the scope of the professional's job. Some cases have taken this view, saying that sex is such an aberration from acceptable practice that it cannot be the basis for a claim based on vicarious liability. For example, one court refused to hold a hospital liable under a claim of *respondeat superior* in a case in which a physician allegedly sexually assaulted a patient he was seeing in the hospital.[4] Other courts have, however, been willing to hold an employer liable for the actions of its employee. In *Marston* v. *Minneapolis Clinic of Psychiatry and Neurology, Ltd.*, the court said that "sexual relations between a psychologist and a patient (were) a well-known hazard and . . . foreseeable and a risk of employment."[5]

Negligent Hiring/Supervision/Retention

The courts seem to be more receptive to claims under this doctrine. An agency can be held responsible if the plaintiff can prove that the agency was negligent in hiring the professional, by, for example, not checking into his past history of exploitation. In the case of *Evan* v. *Huggett*, the church was held responsible for hiring an unfit pastor.[6] In other cases, the court has found that the employee was negligently supervised. There is a widespread view that the Catholic Church quietly and routinely moves priests who have engaged in sexual abuse to another parish, thereby potentially risking the claim that they negligently retained an employee. In *Howard* v. *Roman Catholic Bishop for the Diocese of Stockton*, in response to a police investigation, the diocese promised that the priest would have no further access to children. "The investigation was closed, and O'Grady (the priest) was sent to another parish, where he continues to molest children."[7] In their 1997 supplement, apparently in response to the surge of lawsuits against the clergy, Bisbing et al. (1997) provide suggestions of ways in which employers can avoid liability by undertaking background checks and investigating "red flags" of "possible or probable molesting behavior in the past" (18–21).

Bisbing et al. attempt to expand this basis for a suit by encouraging lawyers to argue that health care employers have a nondelegable duty to "supply a competent staff and to ensure patients' safety" (219). They cite several cases in support of this duty in areas other than professional sexual misconduct. No cases appear to have been decided in the area of professional sexual misconduct based on this duty, but it provides an illustration of efforts to expand the claim by applying related legal concepts.

Spousal Causes of Action

"New" plaintiffs have made claims recently arguing that they have been damaged by the sexual misconduct of the professional. This parallels the trend discussed elsewhere to define the victims more broadly to include third parties, such as family members. The plaintiffs are usually married couples trying to recover against the wife's therapist who had been sexually involved with her. While these cases seek to expand liability, they have ironically often come up against a countermovement to limit the availability of actions based on the marital state. Until recently, common law allowed the husband to sue a third party for what was known as alienation of affections or criminal conversation (a charmingly archaic term for extramarital sexual intercourse) with his wife. Because such actions were seen as illustrative of an inappropriately patriarchal attitude to women as property, many states have abolished them. So when a modern husband has tried to sue his wife's therapist when there has been a sexual relationship, he comes face-to-face with the argument that such actions are no longer available in the law. Even when the claim is not based on alienation of affection or criminal conversation, courts have been reluctant to expand a professional's duty to third parties. In the case of *Homer* v. *Long*, for example, the husband sued his wife's psychiatrist, alleging that he had seduced the wife, thereby causing the breakup of the marriage.[8] Presumably in an attempt to sidestep the abolition of the traditional actions, he based his claim on negligence, fraud, negligent misrepresentation, and intentional infliction of emotional distress. The court denied his claim, arguing that the psychiatrist owed no duty to the husband and that what the husband was actually claiming was recompense for the breakup, which was barred by the abolition of the traditional actions of criminal conversation and alienation of affection.

The only situation in which a spouse has been able to sue a therapist successfully for having a sexual relationship with his wife was a case in which the therapist was treating both husband and wife for marital problems. The court in *Figueredo-Torres* v. *Nickel* held that the husband's claim of negligence and intentional infliction of emotional distress was not barred by the abolition of alienation of affection and criminal conversation because the psychiatrist owed *him* a duty of care as well as his wife because he was also treating the husband.[9]

Posttermination Sex

If the professional relationship has ended, the issue of whether the defendant still owes the plaintiff a duty of care can be complex because the situations can vary so much, especially if the case deals with a professional whose professional organization has not made it clear when the obligation not to have a sexual relationship with a client or patient ends. The issue has been the subject of recent debate in the field. Some professional associations prohibit sexual relations for a specific period of time (e.g., the American Psychological Association prohibits sexual contact between therapists and former patients for two years after termination of therapy), while the American Psychiatric Association prohibits it forever (see Bisbing et al., 1995: 728 for details). The latter policy is premised on the view that there can never be a "normal" relationship once the patient has been in therapy with the therapist and that, therefore, consent is never free of transference issues. From a feminist perspective, the situation presents women with another double bind. Either she is so dependent that she can never make an independent decision, or she is a free agent and needs no protection from the continuing patriarchal power of her therapist.

Suing "New" Defendants

Efforts to apply the law that was so appropriate for therapists to other professionals, like the clergy and lawyers and professors, have encountered some difficulty. The nature of these relationships means that professional sexual exploitation fits less clearly into the framework of malpractice law. We have seen how easily therapists fit into the medical model with its clearly articulated standards of negligence. For nonmedical professionals, the nature of the relationship is more diffuse, and the obligations are less clear-cut.

Nontherapist Professions

Medical Doctors. The issues involved in suing a nonpsychiatric physician are somewhat different, as the claim of transference, so central to negligence, is less easily made. While there is increasing professional agreement that physicians should not engage in sexual behavior with their patients, courts have not yet been enthusiastic about accepting this expanded claim. There is still a sense that a sexual relationship is not negligence but an affair. With such an approach, courts ignore the power imbalance in the doctor–patient relationship in which the patient's ability to "consent" to sex is constrained by her need for medical help and the patriarchal quality of many medical relationships. The Supreme Court has begun to recognize the importance of this power imbalance in another context, that of workplace sexual harassment, by determining that the voluntary nature of the relationship is controlling rather than a determination of whether the plaintiff consented in the sense required under rape laws.[10] Using a voluntary standard takes into consideration the pressures felt by a woman from her superiors in the workplace. Recent statements by the American Medical Association and state medical associations that such behavior violates ethical rules are likely to provide support for an argument that sex during an ongoing medical relationship is as unethical (and therefore negligent) as in the therapeutic relationship (see Bisbing et al., 1995: 142–43).

Clergy. The most extensively publicized cases of professional sexual exploitation in recent years have involved members of the clergy who have been found to abuse their parishioners, both children and adults. Some people have expressed concern that the recent tidal wave of lawsuits might bankrupt the Catholic Church, so extensive does the problem appear to be. Those cases that have gone to court have met with mixed success, though many cases have been quietly settled.

The increase in lawsuits against the church has not been confined to sexual exploitation cases but seems to stem from an increased willingness to hold the church responsible for a variety of alleged wrongs (Jenkins, 1996). One of the reasons for the increase in lawsuits against the church is the fact that courts have recently begun to allow punitive damage awards against churches, as happened in the suit against the diocese of Dallas in 1997[11] (Steinfels, 1997). But in addition, as the *Wall Street Journal* has pointed out, "parishioners simply seem more willing to challenge church authority than in the past, and to do so in court" (Geyelin, 1992: 16B). Doubtless, the increase in lawsuits has been fueled by the changes in statutes of limitations, which are discussed later, since so many of the victims of this wave of cases have been children. It should be noted that, while most of the publicity has been about cases directed at the Catholic Church, it has not been the only denomination to be sued. No denomination appears to have been immune from such suits, and recent defendants have included the Church of Latter-Day Saints and the Hare Krishna (Van Voris, 1998; Godstein, 1998).

The basis of the lawsuits in the case of child sexual abuse by members of the clergy is not a problematic issue. The issue of consent is not relevant here, since children cannot legally consent to sex. It seems that the responsibility of the church is also often clear-cut under the third-party doctrines discussed earlier. Until recently, many churches, most notably the Catholic Church, had a policy of simply removing the abuser from the parish where there had been trouble and placing him elsewhere. To the extent that this was so, the church can now hardly claim ignorance of his behavior. In addition, the application of the doctrine of negligent retention, discussed earlier, is clear.

In the case of claims by adults, however, the legal basis for a claim is less clear-cut. Unlike therapists, no automatic rule makes a sexual relationship between the professional and the client unethical. Whether clergy counselors can be held liable for professional malpractice is still unclear. It is easier in those cases in which the professional is trained in counseling, especially if his training is in one of the recognized counseling disciplines.

There are other legal barriers to a successful claim against the clergy. The doctrine of charitable immunity traditionally protected the church (and other charitable institutions) from suit or limited the amount of its liability. This doctrine has been limited in its scope or abolished altogether in some states but may still provide limitations in the efforts to sue the church (Bisbing et al., 1995: 285). Efforts to avoid the doctrine require that the plaintiff plead a conspiracy, which is not easy (Rubino, 1997).

The First Amendment protection of freedom of religion is another matter of legal concern. It does not protect the clergy from intentional torts, but the issue is less clear in claims of clergy malpractice (see Bisbing et al., 1995: 281). On one hand, it could be argued that an investigation into alleged clergy malpractice would involve an unconstitutional intrusion into religious beliefs and practice. On the other hand, some people argue that a compelling state interest in regulating pastoral counselors overrides the protection of religion in the First Amendment. Recent cases have been decided both ways. For example, in *Bear Valley Church of Christ* v. *DeBose*, the court held that the defense must prove that the conduct in question is motivated by a sincerely held religious belief.[12] Some courts are more reluctant to interfere in religious matters, as was the case in *L.L.N.* v. *Clauder*, in which the court held that claims of negligent supervision in a case of professional sexual misconduct would "require a court to develop a 'reasonable cleric' standard of care which would involve the interpretation of church canons and internal church policies."[13] Efforts to sidestep the problems of the First Amendment in clergy misconduct cases have had some success by arguing that the misconduct is a breach of a fiduciary duty rather than clergy malpractice. In *F.G.* v. *MacDonnell, et al.*, the court said, "The First Amendment does not insulate a member of the clergy from actions for breach of fiduciary duty arising out of sexual misconduct that occurs during a time when the clergy member is providing counseling to a parishioner."[14] In cases like this, it is not necessary to establish a standard of care (with the problems of examining religious doctrine) as in the malpractice claim but, rather, that a parishioner trusted and sought counseling from a pastor. A violation of that trust constitutes a breach of the duty.

Lawyers representing plaintiffs who claim abuse by the clergy have begun to use fraud and coercion as bases for their suits. Such a claim has the benefit of avoiding the statute of limitations problems, discussed later. In the case of *Doe* v. *Kos and Grahmann*, the case against the Catholic diocese mentioned earlier, the jury accepted the plaintiffs' argument that the diocese had, among other things, committed fraud through misrepresentation, concealment, or a failure to disclose. One would not normally think of the clergy as engaged in knowing fraud and deception, but courts are beginning to accept that the church can be judged just like any other defendant, especially given the increasingly assertive defense that lawyers are beginning to mount as their interests change from a concern about public image to protecting their assets and reputation through aggressive defense.

Lawyers. Lawyers have been much slower than other professionals to condemn sexual relations between attorney and client. Indeed, many lawyers still believe that sex between client and lawyer is, at least some of the time, quite acceptable. Bisbing et al. (1995), the "bible" of professional sexual misconduct, has chapters on several professions but none on lawyers. In addition, there is a strong feeling that specific rules against sexual behavior violate attorneys' right to privacy and freedom of association (Firestone and Simon, 1992). The variation of opinion and the fervor with which the different opinions are held can be seen from the recent heated debate around the drafting of ethics rules governing sexual relations with clients in California (Firestone and Simon, 1992; Langford, 1995). The majority of states do not have a specific ethics rule on the subject, although that may be slowly changing. Minnesota, a leader in the professional sexual exploitation movement, is working to pass a law forbidding lawyers from initiating sexual relations with their clients.[15] The Supreme Court of Wisconsin adopted a rule that proscribes sexual contact between attorney and client under specified circumstances (Wis. S.C.R. 20: 1.8[k] Sexual Contact between Lawyers and Clients). The American Bar Association's Standing Committee on Ethics and Professional Responsibility, after examining the issue for the first time in 1992, wrote a formal opinion and issued a nonbinding ethical rule advising against sexual contact between attorney and client (ABA Comm. on Ethics and Professional Responsibility, Formal O. No. 364 [1992]). It stated that a sexual relationship may involve an unfair exploitation of the lawyer's fiduciary position and may impair the lawyer's ability to represent the client.

The difficulty stems from two divergent views of clients: one in which they are simply equals consulting a professional for advice and the other in which they are very like patients who are not equal to the professional but who become dependent and may have feelings very similar to the transference that characterizes therapist–patient relationships (Firestone and Simon, 1992: 682–85). Some writers on the subject are beginning to recognize that not all clients are alike and that the lawyer has a different responsibility depending on the type of client and the nature of the consultation. The divorce client is the classic example of a vulnerable person whose relationship with her lawyer may have many of the characteristics of a therapist–patient relationship. For that reason, the chief judge of New York has imposed a disciplinary rule on divorce lawyers that prohibits sexual relations between a lawyer and a client during the divorce case (Labaton, 1993).

Because there is less consensus about the ethics of lawyer–client sex, it has been more difficult to make successful claims of breach of a duty owed by the lawyer to the client, especially in the absence of some financial loss. If many in the profession believe that sexual relationships between lawyer and client are acceptable, it is difficult to claim a breach of any duty owed by the lawyer to the client as a basis for a lawsuit. In one recent case, for example, the court refused to recognize that having sexual relations with a divorce client was a breach of the attorney's fiduciary duty, in part because the plaintiff did not allege actual damages.[16]

A jury in Rhode Island found that a lawyer had intentionally inflicted emotional distress on the plaintiff, a divorce client, when he coerced her into a sexual relationship.[17] The jury also found that the attorney had committed battery and made fraudulent representations to the plaintiff and awarded her $25,000 in compensatory damages and $200,000 in punitive damages.[18] The case was, however, overturned on appeal on the grounds that the plaintiff had suffered no damage as a result of the legal malpractice, since the attorney's legal representation was said to be "well-performed and successful."[19]

At this stage, it seems that courts are unlikely to hold in favor of a plaintiff who cannot prove that she suffered financial loss as a result of the sexual relationship. If she can prove that the attorney failed to provide "competent legal services" as a result of the sexual contact and that she suffered financially as a result, then she will be successful in her claim of legal malpractice.[20] Otherwise, courts continue to adhere to the view that these relationships are consensual and beyond the scope of legal redress.

Professors. Bisbing et al. (1995) devote a chapter to a discussion of claims against university professors, arguing that while the context is quite different from that of other professional relationships dealt with in the book, the claim is structurally similar (339). As with lawyers, there is a fundamental disagreement within the university community about whether sex between a professor and a student is consensual sex or professional sexual exploitation. This conflict is mirrored in the varying responses of different institutions; some prohibit the behavior in varying circumstances (depending on whether the student is actually taught by the professor), some discourage it, and some have no formal policy at all. Academic institutions seem to be moving in the direction of at least discouraging such behavior, perhaps as a result of recent developments in the law under Title IX of the Education Amendments of 1972, making it easier for plaintiffs to sue for money damages in sexual harassment cases between a professor and a student.

Bisbing et al. (1995) specifically encourage new development by suggesting various bases for lawsuits, though they cite no cases framed in terms of professional sexual misconduct (348–56). Proving negligence could be difficult because standards of care are less clearly articulated between professor and student than those for other professionals discussed in this chapter. The inequality of the relationship and the patriarchal power that infuse the professor–student relationship are similar to other professional relationships. However, those few cases that have been decided have been framed in terms of sexual harassment (where the workplace is also a locus of unequal and potentially coercive relationships) and related employment claims rather than negligence.

Unlicensed Therapists

The cases discussed in the first section of this chapter were against licensed therapists, bound by the licensing and ethics requirements of their profession. In our society, however, it is very easy to practice counseling or therapy without being licensed. As long as one does not pretend to have qualifications or a license that one does not have, it is perfectly legal to hang out a shingle and provide counseling or advice and to call it whatever one wants. Many people do exactly that. Making a claim that the actions of an unlicensed professional violate the standards of acceptable professional behavior is, therefore, more difficult in such cases where there are no generally acceptable professional standards of care. This is especially true if the claim is not only based on the sexual contact but on what otherwise would be considered related boundary violations.

If a therapist says he is qualified and he is not, a plaintiff has an additional basis for a claim of negligence. In the case of *Corgan v. Muehling*, the court agreed with the plaintiff that she had stated a cause of action based on his holding himself out to be qualified and competent, although he was unregistered, and that he was negligent by having sexual relations with his patient and mishandling the transference phenomenon.[21]

If a therapist is unlicensed, he is less likely to be insured and, therefore, a less promising prospect for the payment of damages, though if he works for a clinic, he may be insured through the clinic. In addition, it might also be possible to sue his employer under the doctrines of third-party liability discussed earlier.

Innovative Doctrines Used in Other Contexts

Some lawyers have attempted to take legal doctrines used in altogether different contexts and apply them to professional sexual exploitation. For example, in one case, lawyers for three men who alleged that as children they were sexually exploited by priests attempted to sue the Catholic Church under the federal Racketeer Influenced and Corrupt Organizations Act (RICO).[22] They accused two priests of conspiring "to create a sex ring of children that could be abused by the two Roman Catholic priests, and on information and belief, other priests."[23] Because the case was settled several months later, we will never know whether such a claim would have been successful, although one expert believes that the plaintiffs were "swimming against the tide, because the courts are generally hostile to civil RICO and novel and expansive uses of the statute by private plaintiffs."[24] Bisbing et al. (1995) recognize the possibility of borrowing doctrine from other areas when they describe RICO as well as other remedies as "relatively untraveled avenues in sexual exploitation actions and could prove to be attractive alternatives or supplements to the traditional . . . actions" (173). The other remedies they mention are civil rights suits and consumer fraud statutes. There appear to be no cases directly using either federal or state civil rights remedies as the basis for a claim of professional misconduct. Their usefulness is limited both by the fact that since this is a constitutional remedy, it can be used only in the public context, and by the fact that it would work only in egregious cases, as it requires proof of "gross negligence" or "deliberate indifference." Likewise, some states specifically exclude professionals in their consumer protection statutes, and a further limitation exists in the requirement that the public interest be adversely affected by the claimed sexual exploitation. Women who have been exploited could argue that their sexual exploitation by a professional has negatively affected the public interest since it sets a tone in which such exploitation seems an acceptable risk of seeking help. In appropriate fact situations, all these remedies provide possibilities for innovative plaintiffs' lawyers.[25]

One recent piece of legislation opens up the possibility of a new cause of action in these cases. The Gender Motivated Violence Act (commonly known as the Violence Against Women Act) provides for a civil remedy for victims of violent acts that are motivated by gender. For the Act to apply, the behavior in question has to be a felony under state or federal law, so it could be used only in those states that have made therapist–patient sexual contact a felony, and the plaintiff would have to prove that the crime was motivated, at least in part, by "gender animus" (Bisbing et al., 1999: 16). The statute has been used successfully in at least one case.[26] The constitutionality of the statute has been questioned but has not yet been resolved by the Supreme Court.

CHECKS AND BALANCES: STATUTES OF LIMITATIONS AND INSURANCE

Efforts to expand the law in one direction inevitably lead to counterefforts by those defending such actions who, in their turn, push to limit that expansion. The law applying statutes of limitations provides a good example of the swings of the legal pendulum here, with plaintiffs' lawyers pushing in one direction, defense attorneys in the other, and legislatures and courts responding to both.

Statutes of Limitations

Basic Principles of Statutes

Statutes of limitations exist in all states to limit the period during which a plaintiff can make a claim in tort law. The period, which is usually two to three years from the date of the injury, is intended to protect defendants from the difficulties and unfairness of trying to obtain evidence to defend themselves after a lapse of time. It has always been recognized that such a rule can work to the detriment of the plaintiff, but it is considered to be part of the price to be paid for such protection. When a statute of limitations is

applied to certain types of injury, including professional sexual exploitation, the plaintiff is frequently unable to sue. This is because in some cases,
as we have seen, it takes many years for the victim to realize that she has
been injured, by which time the statute of limitations has long since expired. For many victims, the permutations of the relevant statute of limitations are the major issue in determining the success or failure of their claim.
Finding ways of circumventing these statutes is integral to the work of
plaintiffs' attorneys. How to deal with statutes of limitations is one of the
central threads running through meetings of survivors (e.g., SNAP meeting, 1996; the Linkup meeting, 1997). To survivors it seems unfair and legalistic that of two victims, both of whose claims look similar, one may
succeed in court while the other does not.

Extension of the Doctrine

The extent to which the law bends to protect either the plaintiff or the
defendant changes in response to political attitudes. In the last few
decades, courts have generally become more favorable to plaintiffs in tort
claims, expanding their legal rights in court (Schuck, 1988). It is part of the
victims' rights movement, which has had significant recent success in various legal areas. Expansion of statutes of limitations has broadened the
ability of plaintiffs to bring claims in appropriate cases.

As part of this movement to expand the rights of victims, some states
have "tolled" the statute (meaning that the clock does not begin to run)
until the victim has actually discovered that she has been injured (see
Keeton, 1984: 165). This rule, known as the discovery rule, turns on the judicial interpretation of statutes of limitations, which usually define the
time period as running from the "accrual" of the cause of action (Bisbing
et al., 1995: 692). Courts have generally defined accrual as beginning only
when the victim discovers or should discover that she has been harmed by
the defendant's conduct.

The unlimited use of the discovery rule leads to the opposite inequity
from that which exists in its absence. Instead of leaving meritorious claims
unremedied, it leaves defendants virtually permanently at risk of a claim.
Some cases of professional sexual misconduct, especially by the clergy, are
now being brought that date back to the 1970s and occasionally earlier. For
this reason, there has been an opposite swing of the pendulum in states
that have established special statutes of limitations on medical malpractice
claims or limits on the discovery rule by statutes of "repose," which place
an outer limit on the period of time during which suit can be brought
(Bisbing et al., 1995: 722–24; 1997: 63). Clearly, this is a complex area of the
law, which makes understandable potential plaintiffs' belief in the arcane
and unfair quality of the law.

The combination of these rules as they apply to professional sexual exploitation is illustrated by the Wisconsin statute, which states:

If a person is entitled to bring the action . . . [but] is unable to bring the action due to the effects of the sexual contact or due to any threats, instructions or statements from the therapist, the period of inability is not part of the time limited for the commencement of the action, except that this subsection shall not extend the time limitation by more than 15 years.[27]

Wisconsin's statute, one of the few statutes that deal specifically with the problem of the statute of limitations as it applies to professional sexual exploitation, reaches essentially the same legal result as the cases and statutes that address the issue more generally. Victims are not barred from making a claim by the statute of limitations if they can prove that they realized that they had been harmed only years later (but no more than the outer limit described in the statute) and filed their claim within the required two or three years after that.

So much for the statutes. The way they are interpreted is markedly influenced by perceptions of the salience of the problem. To the extent that professional sexual exploitation is viewed as an injustice in need of a remedy, judges and lawyers may interpret these rules broadly. A lawyer in Minnesota who has been involved with many cases of clergy sexual exploitation, mostly for the defense, said that the oldest case he had related to events that allegedly took place in 1955. "The statutes of limitations rules are useless. You can't get rid of cases on summary judgment because they say that they didn't fully recognize the abuse until last year. That is a question of proof, so you need to go to trial" (Schiltz, 1993). Not surprisingly, plaintiffs' lawyers have a different view. They see the statutes of limitations as an increasing barrier to the success of their claims, especially in cases of clergy sexual misconduct, as the church has begun to defend against claims with more vigor. Plaintiffs' lawyers look for ways to avoid the constraints of the statutes of limitations, particularly in cases of third-party liability. Suits against third parties, most commonly the church, are not included in the discovery rule, which extends the statutes of limitations, thus leaving only a two- or three-year period in which to sue.

In those states that do not have a discovery rule, or where it does not apply, as in the case of third parties, innovative lawyers have relied on the general doctrines of equitable estoppel and fraudulent concealment to extend the time available in which to sue for victims of professional sexual exploitation who take some time to realize they have been harmed. Under equitable estoppel, a plaintiff needs to prove that the defendant had played a role in inducing the plaintiff to postpone bringing suit or concealing a cause of action that would have been available to her. The courts recognize the various ways in which a professional can abuse his power over a vulnerable patient. In the case of *Coopersmith* v. *Gold*, the plaintiff asked her psychiatrist if transference was involved after her first sexual encounter with him.[28] He denied it, and the sexual relationship continued.

The court refused the psychiatrist's request for summary judgment, reasoning that he had falsely advised her that there was no transference in order to exploit her sexually. Under this doctrine, courts essentially say, We don't like what you have done, so we won't let you claim the benefits of the statute of limitations. Similarly, in fraudulent concealment, a plaintiff has to prove that the defendant wrongfully concealed the disputed behavior and that the concealment prevented the plaintiff from discovering the cause of action. As we saw in the case against the diocese of Dallas, the plaintiffs successfully argued that the church knew about the sexual abuse and fraudulently concealed it by engaging in a cover-up (Demarest, 1997).

A third argument, that of religious duress, tried by attorneys to sidestep the statutes in the case of suits against the church, has not yet been successful (Roseman, 1999). They argue that children do not report their abuse until long after it has occurred because they are under duress from the power of the church and the priest, which is an important tenet of Catholic doctrine.

Insurance

Because insurance companies play such a central role in these cases, cases are often settled in circumstances where the plaintiff might not win if the case were to go to trial. In fact, the vast majority of cases of professional sexual misconduct against therapists are settled, even if the legal claim is not airtight (Rubino, 1997). Insurance companies make strategic decisions about the relative attractiveness of both the plaintiff and defendant as well as the merits of the case. Thus, even if the claim is not the strongest, insurance carriers are likely to settle if the plaintiff comes across as a young, vulnerable woman, and the defendant appears to be uncaring or unpleasant. Some defendants refuse to settle despite the advice of the insurance company or their lawyer that there is a strong case against them. For this reason, an examination of the reported cases provides a somewhat distorted view of what is going on in civil lawsuits in the area. By contrast, the church is currently defending clergy sexual misconduct cases with great fervor because of what it sees as challenges to its reputation and autonomy. Issues surrounding the insurance policies of the clergy are therefore different.

The high rate of settlement of therapist sexual misconduct cases has not, however, prevented insurance companies from looking for ways to cut their losses because of the surge of claims. Sexual involvement by psychiatrists with their patients has been described as the second leading cause of all professional practice litigation (Perr, 1989: 212). Another source claimed that sexual misconduct was the single highest category of claims filed under therapist malpractice policies and that these claims represented 56 percent of the total proceeds paid on all claims.[29] Therapists are usually insured for "professional services rendered." Plaintiffs argue that a therapist who has a sexual relationship with his patient is providing negligent professional services, which should be covered by the insurance.

Standard professional insurance policies state that the insurer will pay "all sums which the insured shall become legally obligated to pay as damages arising out of the *performance of professional services* rendered or which should have been rendered during the policy period by the insured." Thus, an insurance carrier may attempt to avoid liability by arguing that sexual misconduct is not part of the professional services rendered. In response to that argument, some courts have said that, indeed, it is "inextricably related to the professional services provided or withheld."[30] The basis for the connection between the sexual conduct and the therapist's professional services is the mishandling of transference and countertransference, which are generally accepted by the profession to be central to the therapeutic relationship.

Insurers have also tried to avoid paying claims for therapists by arguing that it is against public policy to insure for intentional or criminal acts. "If the insured's conduct was criminal, outrageous, or beyond the bounds of human decency . . . policy considerations mitigate against holding the insurer liable for payment of damages and that the insured alone should bear the burden of compensating the injured parties" (Bisbing et al., 1995: 907). The practical problem with this argument is that the professional is much less likely to be able to pay the damages than is his "deep-pocketed" insurer. The argument has not met with much success in the courts either. In one case, the court made an analogy to automobile insurance: "[W]here transference is a treatment phenomenon, it is no more incongruous for the professional liability carrier to insure the therapist against the risk he may not abstain from a sexual relationship with a patient, than it is for the auto liability carrier to insure a driver against the risk he may not abstain from exceeding the speed limit or driving while drunk."[31]

The public policy argument has been used successfully to prevent insurers from limiting coverage in at least one state where insurers tried to deny a claim altogether when sexual misconduct was part of the claim, but other such claims have been less successful[32] (see Bisbing et al., 1995: 914–17; 1997: 85).

Efforts to limit liability by drafting exclusions or caps (limiting the amount they will pay in such cases) into their policies have provided insurance carriers with a better defense to claims of plaintiffs. If the insurer can prove that the defendant's claim is entirely based on the sexual conduct and that such conduct was excluded from coverage, the plaintiff will not prevail in her claim. In the case of *Govar v. Chicago Insurance Co.*, the court held that the essential element of the claim was the sexual conduct. Since that was excluded by the clause that read that "(t)his insurance does not apply to claims arising out of any sexual acts performed by the named insured . . . if such acts occurred as an essential element of the cause of action so adjudicated," the plaintiff failed to recover.[33] Some courts have been more supportive of plaintiffs' claims, as, for example, in *Legion Insurance Co.* v. *Vemuri*, in which the exclusion was for any claim based on undue familiarity. The court concluded that the term "claim" was ambiguous and interpreted it in favor of the insured to refer only to the part of the claim dealing with the sexual misconduct and not the entire claim.[34]

Lawyers acting for plaintiffs in these cases have attempted to get around the exclusions and caps in a variety of ways. They have argued that these exclusions are discriminatory since about 90 percent of the claimants of professional sexual misconduct are women. This disparate impact argument, commonly used in cases of discrimination (some of them dealing with insurance), has not yet been successful in this context. In *American Home Assurance Co.* v. *Cohen*, the court found that nothing prevented different treatment of men and women when there were, as in this situation, significant differences in the risk for which they were insuring, and the policy was neutral on its face.[35] What is called concurrent proximate cause has been more successful against policy limits. Lawyers for plaintiffs argue that the malpractice itself stemmed from acts other than the sexual conduct. Experts maintain that in cases of professional sexual misconduct there is invariably other negligence as well (Jorgenson, Bishing, and Sutherland, 1992). For example, in one case the court found that the therapist's "abuse of the transference process by having sex and his abandonment were each potential proximate causes of (the patient's) psychological injuries."[36] Many sexually exploitative therapists also engage in what are termed boundary violations, including such behavior as socializing with the client, dating her, employing her, having extensive personal phone conversations, or telling her too much about themselves. These boundary violations are considered inappropriate in therapeutic relationships. In addition, the termination of the relationship, which may be connected in some way to the sexual relationship, can often be proven to have been mishandled, another basis for a claim of negligence other than the sexual exploitation.

Insurance also plays a role in efforts to claim for professional sexual exploitation in other professions. In the case of professional sexual exploitation by therapists, most courts see the malpractice growing out of transference, which is not a central element in other professional relationships. Accordingly, when the professional sexual misconduct of other professions is at issue, courts generally accept defendants' arguments that the sexual behavior is intentional or criminal and, therefore, not a legitimate part of the professional services for which the professional was insured. However, if the plaintiff suing a nontherapist physician can argue that the professional was, in fact, providing therapy to the patient, she might be able to recover under his malpractice insurance.[37]

Some scholars have argued that transference should be extended to relationships with nontherapist professionals in which there is an imbalance of power, which would bring claims under malpractice insurance coverage (see Bisbing et al., 1995: 937–40). This view would provide a remedy for a woman who seeks professional help in a relationship of trust who is otherwise punished by the legal definition of a therapeutic versus a nontherapeutic relationship. A woman seeking help does not define her relationship with a professional as either therapeutic or nontherapeutic. To her, the professional is someone she trusts and who seems responsive to her needs, and the relationship is not dependent on the nature of his credentials and the details of his insurance policy, which guide her chances of legal recovery.

In the case of clergy sexual misconduct, insurance issues present a complex and confused picture. Like many other aspects of this issue, the church is reluctant to divulge the nature of its relationship with insurers. At the 1997 Linkup conference, attendees shared rumors about the Catholic Church's insurance arrangements, but even those who were professionally involved in lawsuits were unable to present a clear picture. In some cases, the church appears to be self-insured, while in others, it has had less than satisfactory relationships with its insurers during the spate of claims in the last decade or so. More than one lawyer has stressed that they are not interested in the insurance arrangements, as they look to church property to satisfy the judgments they obtain (Demarest, 1997; Rubino, 1997).

APPLICATION OF EXISTING STATUTES

In some states, statutes that existed before professional sexual misconduct came to the attention of the law or were passed with a broader purpose can be applied. These statutes have, however, been of limited utility, as they do not usually cover the facts of professional sexual misconduct.

Criminal Statutes

Rape Laws

In general, ordinary rape statutes will not apply in professional sexual exploitation cases because of the issue of consent. Attempts to apply rape laws are based on the belief that the victim cannot be said to have freely consented to a sexual relationship with the professional because of transference, dependence, and vulnerability. This view, however, does not generally prevail. As has been well documented in the rape literature, courts apply traditionally male ideas of the nature of consent (see, e.g., Estrich, 1987). This requirement of consent is a particularly heavy burden in cases of professional sexual exploitation. Not only has the woman been social-ized to be passive and acquiescent in general, but she is in a vulnerable state in particular need of the help and support of the professional she has consulted. The fact that the professional is in a position of power is rarely factored into a determination of whether she consented or not. One no-table exception that can be applied in cases of professional sexual ex-ploitation is Wyoming's statute that makes it a crime for someone in a position of authority to abuse his power to obtain sex.[38] Feminist legal scholarship has begun to make the argument to extend the law in force in Wyoming to all rape law. Stephen J. Schulhofer (1998) argues in his book *Unwanted Sex* that the law is too narrowly focused on whether the defen-dant uses force or violence, rather than intimidation or coercion. He frames an argument around the abuse of power, which would bring into rape law those who use their power as professionals to coerce women into having sex with them. This appears to be a very typical scenario in cases of professional–client sex. In one study of a clinical population, Luepker (1999) found that 95 percent of her sample were coerced into having sex.

Even in those cases where the physician has misled his patient into be-lieving that the sex was part of the treatment, courts have not always found him guilty of rape despite the existence of statutes that criminalize sexual conduct when consent was fraudulently obtained (Jorgenson, Randles, and Strasberger, 1991: 666). While such an assertion may seem outlandish to some, Luepker's study found that 56 percent of her sample reported that the practitioner used "therapeutic deception" in which he argued that the sex would be therapeutic or, in the case of clergy, "God's will."

It is easier to obtain a conviction in those unusual cases where, for ex-ample, the physician has administered drugs before engaging in sex with his patient both because the court is more willing to acknowledge the lack of consent (as traditionally defined) and because many states have statutes that specifically declare such behavior to fall within the definition of rape. In one case the doctor used both electroconvulsive shock therapy and drugs to make his patients helpless before sexually assaulting them. Here the court had no difficulty convicting him of rape and incarcerating him.[39]

With the changes in the rape laws over the last 20 years, some develop-ments are relevant here. Many states now include in their rape statutes provisions that sexual acts with a person suffering from serious mental impairment are criminal. While this, on the face of it, should be applica-ble to cases of professional sexual exploitation, courts have been reluctant to apply these statutes to any cases except the most egregious ones (Jor-genson, Randles, and Strasberger, 1991: 667). So these laws do not add significantly to the legal arsenal available to the victim of professional sexual exploitation.

There have been a few efforts to confront the issue directly. Several states have specifically defined sexual contact or assault under the guise of treatment as rape (Bisbing et al., 1995: 839). These statutes cover those cases in which the physician convinces the patient that he is treating her when, in fact, he is assaulting her. This happens more often than one might expect, but the statute does not cover the typical case, where there is no *specific* deception. Cases where the therapist said something generally about the sex being good for the patient's psyche, rather than an expressed or implied indication that it was a specific medical treatment, are not likely to result in conviction. The statutes are also directed only at those who provide medical treatment, although one court has indicated that it will apply such statutes to psychotherapists.[40]

Legislation Specific to Professional Sexual Misconduct

Specific Criminal Statutes

As we have seen, efforts to use either traditional criminal statutes or even newer statutes that were not designed to deal with the case of professional sexual exploitation have not been very effective. For this reason, among others, there have been efforts to pass laws specifically designed for professional sexual misconduct. These laws are discussed in detail in the next chapter.

Civil Statutes

Several states have recently enacted statutes that provide for civil liability for professional sexual exploitation (Bisbing et al., 1998). While, as we have discussed, it is quite possible to sue under the general common law, these statutes make it easier in several ways. They make sexual exploitation negligence per se and create an irrebuttable presumption of a duty of care. In addition, they deal with several issues not covered by common law. For example, Minnesota has amended its statute to extend the statute of limitations to six years from the time the patient knows or has reason to know that the sexual exploitation caused the injury.[41] These statutes also cover the difficult issue of remedies for the former patient by extending the period during which a victim can sue for up to two years after the termination of therapy (Bisbing et al., 1995: 163–64). Some statutes clarify and extend the circumstances when an employer can be liable for the exploitation of the employee (Jorgenson, Randles, and Strasberger, 1991: 710–12). The statutes deal with sexual misconduct of therapists, though that is broadly defined to include a wide range of counseling relationships; some specifically include clergy in pastoral relationships. An important benefit of the statutes is that plaintiffs who use them are protected from the classic (now limited in criminal cases) inquiry into their past sexual history. Without this protection, many victims are fearful of the harassment involved in filing a claim against their therapist, who is in a position to exploit his intimate knowledge of her history. The victim is protected from the revelation of private information both at complaint hearings and at the court trial. These victim-shield statutes do not, however, apply during the victim's civil trial, when damages are at issue. By suing to recover for damages she suffered at the hands of the defendant, the victim has waived her right of confidentiality, so she can no longer be protected from the revelation of private information that the professional has obtained during the confidential relationship.

Without the protections offered by the special civil statutes, defendants in civil claims have used the past history of the plaintiff as evidence of her unreliability and promiscuity to discredit her and negate her claim. As has been clearly documented in the rape literature, this represents the law's perception of "woman as whore," who is assumed to have consented to the sexual activity because she has consented to sex in the past (Tong, 1984). The risk of having her private life paraded before the court is one of the reasons some women choose not to sue in states without the special civil laws.

Mandatory Reporting

The model for mandatory reporting laws is that of child abuse reporting statutes, which have been widely adopted (Nelson, 1984). Experts in the field differ on whether public policy is served by requiring the subsequent therapist of a victim of professional sexual exploitation to report his or her colleague to the appropriate authorities. Research indicates that a very small proportion of those who are sexually exploited report their abuse (Pope and Bouhoutsos, 1986; *Task Force on Sexual Abuse of Patients*, 1991). Requiring a therapist to report could increase those rates. On the other hand, many therapists believe that a reporting requirement interferes with the therapeutic relationship, especially among this population, whose ability to trust has been severely hampered by the exploitation. Some states have tried to compromise by having a rule that allows the patient to decide whether to file a report, after the therapist provides (as required by the statute) a brochure that describes the rights and remedies of the patient.[42] Only Minnesota, the "tough" state on this issue generally, mandates that a subsequent therapist report the name of the abusing therapist once it is known, even if the victim objects (Schoener et al., 1989d: 562–65).

CONCLUSION

The direction of legal development has much to do with which analogies are the most persuasive to courts and legislatures. For example, in the case of professional sexual exploitation the extension of the statutes of limitations seems to have resulted from its being analogized to incest and child sexual abuse. These problems have recently been recognized as being of major concern and as a result have received significant national attention. Not only has the problem been revealed to be widespread, but many cases have come to light only when adults have discovered in therapy or through other means that they were subjected to sexual abuse as children. The recognition that a child can be harmed and become aware of it only in adulthood can be extended to a recognition that an adult can be harmed and not recognize the harm until sometime later. This new understanding is then incorporated in the law in changes in statutes of limitations, first in incest cases and then by analogy in cases of professional sexual exploitation (see Jorgenson and Randles, 1991 for a discussion of appropriate analogies). Publicity about cases in which these recovered memories of child sexual abuse have been found to be untrue has, in turn, triggered a movement back toward a more restricted approach to statutes of limitations. Child abuse also provided the analogy for the mandatory reporting laws in several states. Here the public policy role of professionals in protecting children is extended to patients, who are also seen as vulnerable members of society.

Other analogies have been used in expanding claims in this area. Courts have used the analogy of the fiduciary obligation most commonly seen in the law of trusts to professional sexual misconduct. The case of *Roy* v. *Hartogs* illustrates an early use of the analogy: the court held that the therapist owed his patient a fiduciary obligation analogous to the guardian–ward relationship.[43]

The extension of the concept of transference to professionals other than therapists represents another framing analogy, which was discussed earlier with reference to other professionals. In certain types of attorney–client relationships, for example, the analogy is to that of therapist–patient in their dependence, vulnerability of the client, and power imbalance between the attorney and client, though so far the courts have not generally accepted this analogy.

All of the framing efforts discussed in this chapter have been within the legal system itself. As we have seen, it has been a matter of fitting the "new" problem into the existing legal system, based on the assumption that the legal system is a suitable place to provide redress for claimants. Very few of these efforts have been directed to changing the basic structure of the patriarchal nature of the legal system. Alternative systems of redress that are not part of the current legal system are not suggested by those directly involved in filing legal claims.

Elsewhere in this book, I show that professional sexual contact can be framed in a variety of ways: for example, as a gender issue, as a health issue, or as an issue of abuse of power. Within the legal system, it is framed as a tort issue (one of professional malpractice) or a criminal issue.

Framing professional sexual misconduct as a legal problem forces the claims-makers to fit the claim into the particular confines of a legal claim.

This emphasizes aspects of the claim that might not be considered central by the victim herself or by those who make the claim outside the legal system. It may even be viewed as a distortion of the "real" picture. The most obvious example of this is the redefinition of the problem as one involving boundary violations that are not sexual so that insurance companies can be made to pay the damages. It can also result in the de-emphasizing of the gendered nature of the claim, as the law generally avoids such a focus. As part of the general neglect of professional sexual misconduct as a social problem, feminist scholarship in general and feminist legal scholarship in particular have also ignored it.

A further difficulty with the current legal approach also neglects to place the issue of power in the central position where it belongs. Feminist scholars have had some success in reframing rape as an issue of violence and power, rather than sex. These issues of power may be more subtle but more important in the case of professional sexual misconduct than in rape generally. The power of the professional over the vulnerable help-seeker provides an additional layer to the power of the rapist over his victim. As long as the law does not recognize these layers of power and their legal implications, women continue to be punished for seeking the help they need.

While fitting the claim into the existing legal system may provide a remedy for those individual plaintiffs who file civil lawsuits, it does very little to reconceptualize the problem in a general sense. Seeing the claims as "just like" other forms of malpractice or criminal behavior does very little to change our view of the issue in a more radical way. Without the general guidance of a theoretical framework, each claim is an individual problem rather than an example of a problem that needs to be handled on a group level. The individual case can be connected with the larger issue only through the deterrent value of publicity. This individual legal approach is a quintessential American response to a social problem.

It is also largely an unquestioned response. Much of the focus of the organizations discussed in Chapter 5 is on individual legal claims. Activists do not discuss whether individual lawsuits are the most effective way of effecting social change. In fact, activists see legal victories as the one bright light in an otherwise depressing scene.

Deciding whether these legal developments have been a success depends on the goal. If the goal is for the individual plaintiff, it is easy to decide whether it has been a success or not; she either wins the lawsuit or does not. But in the law, even a verdict in favor of the defendant in a particular case can pave the way for success by future plaintiffs using similar arguments.

Despite the promise of precedent and even failed arguments, the success of a legal framing of the problem is always individual. Its benefits in a broader sense are therefore only indirect. That does not mean that they are not potentially powerful; people and institutions may respond to a threat of legal action and attendant costs where claims based on moral grounds may fail. As we have seen, many activists believe in the power of the law, especially in clergy abuse, to a greater extent than they do in the power of the church to respond to their claims of clergy sexual abuse. Likewise, many of those abused by therapists believe the law to be more likely to substantiate their claim than professional associations or licensing authorities.

It is, of course, hard to measure the accuracy of these beliefs. The scholarly research does not provide much support for the view that the courts can initiate social change (see Rosenberg, 1991). As part of a broader public policy program, the courts can play a significant role. The problem in this case is that there has not been much of a public policy program in this area. Whether the threat of legal action in this context is more effective in changing individual behavior is also unclear. Some anecdotal evidence suggests that some professionals are deterred, though others appear to be impervious to threats, legal or otherwise.

NOTES

1. The remainder of the chapter is by no means an exhaustive treatment of the law but rather is intended to highlight ways in which the law is adapted to encompass a "new" problem.

2. 366 N.Y.S. 2d 297 (Civ. Ct. 1975).

3. For a detailed discussion of this whole issue, see Jorgenson, Randles, and Strasburger (1991: 691–96).

4. *Hoover* v. *University of Chicago Hospital* 51 Ill. App. 3d 263, 368 N.E. 2d 925 (1977).

5. 329 N.W. 2d 306 (Minn. 1982), at 311.

6. Cal. Ct. App. 1992.

7. 28768/275237 (Super. Ct., San Joaquin Co., Calif.), reported in *National Law Journal* (24 August 1998): A8; quote from Jeffrey Anderson, attorney for the plaintiffs.

8. 599 A. 2d 1193 (Md. App. 1992).

9. 584 A. 2d 69 (Md. Ct. App. 1991).

10. *Meritor Savings Bank* v. *Vinson* 477 U.S. 57 1986.

11. That suit was finally settled after the trial for a total of $36.4 million, the largest settlement in a case of this kind. The payment was shared by the diocese and its insurer (Demarest, 1999).

12. 928 P. 2d 1315 (Colo. 1996).

13. 563 N.W. 2d 434 (1997).

14. 696 A. 2d 697 (1997).

15. So far there is a bar association-proposed rule, which must be endorsed by the larger House of Delegates and approved by the Supreme Court (*National Law Journal*, 18 October 1993): 6.

16. *Suppressed* v. *Suppressed* 565 N.E. 2d 101 (Ill. 1990).

17. "Woman Wins Suit on Coerced Affair with Lawyer," *New York Times*, 29 November 1992: 38.

18. Personal interview with plaintiff's attorney, Bart Molloy, 11 June 1993, who described a deluge of telephone calls after the case was written up in the newspaper.

19. *Vallinoto* v. *Sandro* 688 P 2d 830 (1997).

20. *Suppressed* v. *Suppressed* 114.

21. 574 N.E.602 (Ill. 1991)

22. "Lawsuit by Priest Charges Sex Abuse," *New York Times*, 11 June 1993: A17.

23. Ibid.

24. Ibid.

25. For details of the way such remedies would be framed, see Bisbing et al. (1995: 173–78).

26. *Palazzolo* v. *Ruggiano* 993 F.Supp.45 (D.R.I. 1998).

27. Wis. Stat. Ann. s 893.585(2) (West Supp. 1989).

28. 568 N.Y.S. 2d 250 (N.Y. A.D. 3 Dep't 1991).

29. Cited in an unpublished case, *American Home Assurance Co.* v. *Oraker*. Colo. Dist. Ct. No. 90CV6483, 5 Mar. 1992.

30. *St. Paul Fire & Insurance Co.* v. *Love* 459 B.W.2d 698 (Minn. 1990), 700.

31. Ibid., 702.

32. Colorado Title 10 Insurance C.R.S. 10-4-110.3 (1997).

33. *Govar* v. *Chicago Insurance Co.* 879 F.2d 1582 (8th Cir. 1989).

34. 1997 U.S. Dist. LEXIS 19030.

35. 864 F. Supp. 767 (N.D. Ill. 1994).

36. *Cranford Insurance Co.* v. *Allwest Insurance Co.* 645 F. Supp. 1440 (N.D. Cal. 1986), 1444.

37. For example, *Dillon* v. *Callaway* 609 N.E.2d (Ind. Ct. App. 1993).

38. Wyo. Stat. s 6-2-303(a)(vi)(1988).

39. *Eberhart* v. *State* 134 Ind. 651, 34 N.E. 637 (1893).

40. *State* v. *von Klock* 121 N.H. 697, 433 A.2d 1299 (1981).

41. 1989 Minn. Laws 190 s.2.

42. For example, as required in California. Cal. Bus. & Prof. Code s728 (West 1990).

43. 366 N.Y.S. 297 (N.Y. Civ. Ct. 1975) at 299.

—7—

THE CRIMINAL LEGISLATION

We have tried self-regulation using ethics codes, licensing boards, civil codes for over two thousand years. That is long enough to try any plan, and if that doesn't work we need to try something else.
—Schoener, 6 November 1995

INTRODUCTION

This is the rallying cry of those who have been working to pass legislation to criminalize professional sexual misconduct. It represents the frustration many activists feel about the inadequacy of the other methods of controlling this behavior. At last count, 14 states have criminal laws covering the sexual behavior of therapists with their patients, clients, or former patients (Bisbing et al., 1999: 18–20).[1] See Table 7.1 for a list of the statutes. Several other states are currently working on similar statutes, while a total of 9 others have tried but so far have been unsuccessful in their efforts to pass legislation.

The move to criminalize professional sexual exploitation began in 1975, when Masters and Johnson suggested it in an address before the American Psychiatric Association (Masters and Johnson, 1976). The first state to heed this call was Wisconsin, which passed a statute in 1983 (Section 940.22 Stats.), followed by Minnesota in 1985 (Section 297, Minnesota Laws, 1985). The statutes vary as to exactly who and what are covered, as well as whether the offense is a misdemeanor or a felony. Some statutes distinguish between sexual contact and penetration; some define therapy more or less broadly (e.g., whether they include counseling or treatment of drug and alcohol abuse); some include only behavior in a treatment session, while others prohibit sexual contact regardless of where it occurred; some include only current patients, while others include former patients either for a specified period after the termination of therapy or as long as there is emotional dependence on the therapist (Bisbing et al., 1995: 841–51).

Table 7.1
States That Have Criminalized Therapist/Patient Sex and Year of First Statute

Wisconsin	1983
Minnesota	1985
North Dakota	1987
Colorado	1988
California	1989
Maine	1989
Georgia	1990
Iowa	1992
New Hampshire	1992
South Dakota	1993
New Mexico	1993
Connecticut	1993
Arizona	1994
Texas	1995

Most of the research on the legislative process has focused on federal legislation (Kingdon, 1995). Those few studies focusing on state legislation have involved well-publicized national trends that have resulted in widespread legislation in virtually all of the states (e.g., Nelson, 1984; Jacob, 1988). Research has also focused on successful cases, to the neglect of the many efforts to pass legislation that have failed.

Scholars have argued that a number of characteristics are necessary for the passage of legislation, because the barriers to successful policy making are immense (Kingdon, 1995). The issue should be one of national political importance or be on the mass agenda. We have seen in earlier chapters that professional sexual misconduct is not what Nelson describes as a "valence" issue in which everyone can agree that there is a big problem about which "something must be done." Nelson's case study of the widespread adoption of child abuse reporting statutes makes it clear that the perception of the problem as a valence issue was crucial to the success of the movement (Nelson, 1984). Not only is therapist–patient sex not a valence issue, but we know that there is not even any general awareness of the nature of the problem among the public. Other factors that are absent here are also considered central by scholars in the field. The issue is supported by few people in government and has very few spokespeople involved (Kingdon, 1995). We know that social movement organizations are not involved in mobilizing resources for legislative change (Gamson, 1990; Morris, 1984). So, if the efforts to pass legislation to criminalize professional sexual misconduct do not follow the pattern prior research has shown to be necessary, how, then, did the legislation pass, and why did it succeed in some states and not others? The next section examines these questions by describing how the criminal legislation to prohibit professional sexual misconduct did pass in those states that were successful and what happened in those states that failed to pass legislation.

THE LEGISLATIVE PROCESS

How Did the Process Begin?

Interviews with a wide variety of people involved in the efforts to pass legislation show that there are several different patterns for the initiation of legislative efforts. For example, in Wisconsin, the first state to pass criminal legislation prohibiting therapist–patient sex, the chair of the Judiciary Committee was watching the *Phil Donahue Show* in a hotel room. One of the guests had been sexually exploited by her therapist. The legislator decided then and there that "something should be done about it" (Schoener, 1989c: 529).

In New Mexico a therapist was charged with 14 counts of sexual abuse of male Hispanic teenage victims (Noel and Foote, 1994). The therapist who was charged was very well known. He was the past president of the state psychological association, active in the American Psychological Association, and chief of psychology in one of the major HMOs. At around the same time, the newspapers also reported a case of three women victimized during their prelicensure supervision. A third case involved a woman psychologist and three female victims. In addition, there was also an unusually high number of priests whose criminal sexual abuse cases exploded into the public arena after the efforts to have legislation passed had begun. New Mexico is home to a treatment program where priests have long been sent after being involved in sexual misconduct in other states. Their sex abuse cases followed the priests and contributed to the publicity on the issue. All this publicity about all these cases prompted the New Mexico Psychological Association to decide that criminal legislation was needed and to begin efforts to have it passed.

In Iowa one case of therapist–patient sex was on the front page of a local paper for two weeks. The woman who had been sexually exploited used the publicity about her own case to gather together other survivors and activists to lobby for legislation. She went to the chair of the Judiciary Committee, who already knew about her case, to ask that "something be done" (France, 1996).

In half the states where legislative efforts were successful (seven), a high-profile case attracted attention to the issue. As the example of New Mexico shows, sometimes several cases caught the public's attention. By contrast, there were generally no high-profile cases in those states that tried and failed to pass legislation.

For some of the successful states, a high-profile case was not the only way the process began; legislators and other public officials initiated the legislative process in six states (four legislators, two public officials). Survivors of therapist–patient sex were the precipitating force in a further three cases and professional organizations in two. What is notable is the fact that in several states, a single survivor acted as the trigger, as in the Iowa case. In Georgia a survivor persuaded the lawyer representing her in her civil suit to write a letter to the legislature; she herself organized a letter-writing campaign to legislators (Sappington, 1996).

Elite Support

In California the impetus for the initial legislation came from the State Board of Behavioral Science Examiners, the legislative committee that controlled matters of professional licensing. The bill was introduced by the chairman of the Business and Professional Committee, which was responsible for issues of professional misconduct. In North Dakota several legislators with good reputations in the state sponsored the bill, and the executive director of the state medical association was also involved. In the majority of states (11) that were successful, elite support played some role, most often in sponsoring the bill and/or lobbying others to support it. Failures also had elite support in five cases, but it was weaker, especially in the power of the particular legislator who introduced the bill.

Opposition

In seven of the successful states, there was organized opposition to the proposed legislation, in some states from more than one source. Not surprisingly, most of it came from the professional organizations whose members would be affected by the legislation. The medical association was opposed to the legislation in four states, the clergy of various denominations in three, the state psychological association in one, the state psychiatric association in one, and the governor in two. This opposition was overcome in various ways before the legislation was passed.

In the states that failed to pass criminal legislation, there was opposition in all but one state, again from more than one source. Legislators were outspoken in their opposition in three states (in two of them, the legislator who was opposed was the chairman of the Judiciary Committee), powerful lawyers in two, psychiatrists in one, the medical association in one, the Catholic Conference in one, the insurance lobby in one, and the local American Civil Liberties Union (ACLU) in one. This opposition was stronger and better organized than in the successful states and therefore less easy to overcome.

Tactics Used

Both the successful states and those where the legislation failed used the usual tactics in their efforts to pass the legislation. These ranged from testifying at hearings, lobbying legislators, obtaining information from other states, conducting a study, mobilizing the media, organizing a task force and public meetings, arranging a letter-writing campaign. In the states that failed to pass legislation there were simply fewer of the various tactics used, especially testifying and lobbying.

Task Forces

In about half of the successful states, there was some kind of task force (initiated either by the state or by private groups). The task forces, especially those sponsored by the legislature, were able to gather information about the scope of the problem, testify at hearings, help draft the bill, organize publicity, and generally engage in a variety of the tactics described earlier to help pass the legislation. In addition, they provided needed credibility by attesting to the seriousness of the issue.

The existence of a task force did not guarantee success, however. In four of the states that failed to get the legislation passed, there were task forces (two of them sponsored by the legislature), and in the case of New York (also a failure state), there was both a government-sponsored task force and a private one at different times.

Organizations

In both the successful and the unsuccessful states, a number of organizations were involved in the effort to pass the legislation. In both successes and failures, the organization most frequently involved was the state psychological association (in six successful states and three unsuccessful states). In several states the legislation was actually initiated by that organization. Other organizations involved in successful states were other professional groups (three states), churches, women's groups, sexual assault groups, survivor support groups, and human rights groups. In the failures, women's groups tried to have the legislation passed in three states, sexual assault groups in two states, a coalition of eight professional groups in one state, and a church in another. In none of the states, however, either successful or not, were organizations involved whose specific focus was professional sexual misconduct.

Length of Time from Introduction to Passage

For 11 of the successes, the bill passed the first time it was introduced; for two states, it took two years. This is somewhat deceptive, however. In Minnesota, for example, where the legislation passed the first year, the path had been smoothed by a legislatively appointed task force that held hearings over a period of three years. In New Mexico the task force took two years, as did the passage of the bill. California took the longest time for passage: six years. In general, however, the speed with which these states succeeded in getting the law passed stands in marked contrast with that found in other research; for example, Glick (1992) found that it took an average of seven years to pass living will legislation, with two years being the shortest period. For the failures, it is much harder to assess the passage of time; it can be noted, however, that Massachusetts first set up a House committee as long ago as 1989, while most of the others have been trying for at least two or three years and plan to continue or renew their efforts.

Media Publicity

In very few states did the legislation receive widespread publicity. There were only three states in which informants described "quite a lot" of publicity or "several" articles in local newspapers. Only in New Mexico was successful media publicity seen as a strategy to "humanize" the issue in order to make the legislation more likely to pass. By contrast, in Connecticut those involved in working for the passage of the legislation purposely shunned publicity with a view to minimizing the risk that any publicity would trigger objections to the proposed statute.

APPLYING THE THEORY

Much of the research in legislative policy making cannot be applied to this case, as it focuses on issues that are made part of either the public agenda or the government agenda or both (Kingdon, 1995). The issue of professional sexual misconduct has never been part of the public agenda, nor has it been part of the formal agenda.

Scholars have described policies that are controversial, of low salience, and likely to generate organized opposition as "fragile" policies that they argue may take a long time to be translated into legislation because legislators may want to distance themselves from them (Savage, 1985). Criminalizing professional sexual misconduct certainly fits into this category because it has generated organized opposition by powerful groups, while having low public salience. According to the theory, this combination of factors would ensure that it would take a long time for legislation to be passed; yet we have seen that some of the states were able to pass the statute in the first year it was proposed.

The interstate communication that scholars of policy innovation consider important for the passage of legislation has, indeed, had a place in the passage of these statutes, but it has not been of the traditional kind (Glick, 1992). It has not come from the federal government or from national organizations that focus specifically on the issue. In fact, as we have seen, there has been no input from the social movement organizations on this issue; the most that can be said is that a few members have acted individually, with the encouragement of the organization. In general, there has been little of the organizational support that resource mobilization theorists see as central to the process of action for change (Gamson, 1990; Morris, 1984). The relevant national groups, the professional organizations, have usually had no view of the issue or are at least ambivalent about the legislation (e.g., American Psychiatric Association, 1993).

The most important form of communication has, in fact, come from the Walk-In Counselling Center in Minnesota, which has been in the forefront of this movement since it was first framed as a social problem. Largely because of the work of this clinic, Minnesota was the first state to pass a statute making professional sexual misconduct a felony, and other states have used its statute as a model. The center has also been an essential source of advice for activists proposing criminal legislation all over the country.

Scholars have argued that policy innovation follows a pattern in which certain states are seen as leaders (either in general or on specific issues) and are usually in the forefront of innovative legislation. California, Colorado, New York, New Jersey, Oregon, Pennsylvania, Massachusetts, and Wisconsin are the states that are usually early innovators (Glick, 1992). While some of these states were, indeed, early innovators, some of them have been the worst failures. Wisconsin was the first state to pass a law criminalizing therapist–patient sex, with California and Colorado following, though not without difficulty in the case of California. In contrast, New York, Oregon, Pennsylvania, and Massachusetts have tried and failed to pass the legislation, while New Jersey has apparently not tried.

Scholars have also stressed the connection between variables of state partisanship and ideology and successful legislative efforts. Liberal states are considered more fertile ground for innovative legislation, while the opposite is true for conservative states. This connection also fails to explain why some states have succeeded while others have failed, and still others have not even tried. Erikson et al. (1993) have applied this theory by ranking states on the variables of state partisanship and ideology; these rankings show that North Dakota (the third state to pass a law criminalizing therapist–patient sex) is ranked the third most conservative state in the nation, closely followed by two other states that have passed legislation

(South Dakota and Texas). Massachusetts, on the other hand, which has consistently failed in its efforts to pass legislation criminalizing therapist–patient sex, is ranked as the most liberal state, after the District of Columbia. Thus, it is clear that this legislation cannot be accounted for by traditional measures of state conservatism or liberalism.

Resource mobilization theorists predict that states with more "open" polities would be more likely to pass legislation (Jenkins, 1983). While it is difficult to measure openness, one possible indicator might be the nature of the political culture in a particular state. Elazar (1984) classifies political cultures into three major types: traditional, moralistic, and individualistic. Given the characteristics he ascribes to the different political cultures, it appears that the moralistic culture is the most open and the traditional the least, with the individualistic in the middle. He classifies all the states into one of these three categories or into a combination of two cultures.

Using Elazar's model, we find some association between the political culture and the success of this legislation, which is seen in Table 7.2. Of the 9 states classified as moralistic, 5 have passed legislation, while of the 4 classified as traditional, none have. Of those 8 states Elazar considers predominantly moralistic, with a strong individualistic strain (the next most "open" category), 4 have passed legislation. Of the 10 states described as predominantly traditional, with an individualistic strain, 3 have passed legislation. Thus, of the most "open" states, 9 of 17 have passed legislation, while only 3 of the 14 least "open" states did so.

Table 7.2
States That Passed Legislation by Type of Political Culture

Moralistic	MI	Traditional	TI
VT	NH*	VA	TX*
ME*	IA*	SC	OK
MI	KS	MS	NM*
WI*	CA*	TN	WV
ND*	MT		KY
OR	SD*		FL
UT	ID		AL
CO*	WA		GA*
MN*			AK
			LA

MI: Moralistic dominant, strong individualistic strain.
TI: Traditional dominant, strong individualistic strain.

*: Has passed legislation.

Resource mobilization theorists would also argue that the degree to which the opposition is mobilized is an important factor in determining the success of the movement. In this case study, the nature of the mobilization efforts was a more powerful predictor of success or failure than other variables such as ideology, including the mobilization of the opposition. Those states that managed to deal with their opposition did so by organizing lobbying efforts, especially by survivors, redrafting the laws to take into account the objections of those opposed or obtaining publicity that served to frame the opposition in negative terms (e.g., New Mexico, where opposing psychiatrists were made to look as if they opposed the victims in all the well-publicized cases). In several states, the clergy opposed the bill but were either brought into the process and later supported it (e.g., New Mexico) or were "appeased" by the reassurance of a state legislator (Texas). In some states, the opposition of the clergy was addressed by drafting the bill narrowly enough so that it did not generally apply to the clergy; in Georgia, a later bill that would have included the clergy failed because of their opposition. Likewise, legislation failed to pass in Pennsylvania because proponents could not successfully counter the objections of the organized and powerful Catholic Church.

Those involved in attempts to have the legislation passed have, in some cases, tried to do what Jacob (1988) reports was so successful in the case of divorce reform: to define the legislation as routine or, as several of my interviewees called it, a "no-brainer." Including the issue as part of a package involving a more salient issue, either of medicine (Texas), licensing (Colorado), general criminal legislation (Connecticut), or domestic violence (New Hampshire), seems to have helped its passage in several states.

Tactics used to obtain passage of the bills were conventional institutional tactics. There were no marches, no rallies, no disruptions in any of the states, either successes or failures. In general, there was very little support from social movement organizations, a fact that challenges resource mobilization theory. The social movement organizations involved were professional, such as psychological associations, or focused on providing some related service (e.g., rape crisis centers). But these organizations were not usually key players in success cases; they were more likely to have initiated the efforts, which were then picked up by legislators or individual survivors.

In a number of states, a single survivor played a central role in the passage of the legislation, while in others there was a small, unorganized group of survivors without any connection to an organization. Survivors undertook a variety of lobbying tasks, the most important of which was providing a voice for those harmed by professional sexual misconduct. The power of the testimony of an individual survivor cannot be underestimated. In more than one state, one survivor seems to have single-handedly been able to swing the issue by her efforts in the legislature. Many of those

interviewed stressed how important it was to have legislators hear specifically from those who had suffered professional sexual exploitation. In some
cases, survivors testified at public hearings; in others, to the judiciary committee or to the legislature as a whole. In Iowa one survivor told me
proudly, "I spoke to 123 of the 150 members of the legislature, either individually or in groups of two or three" (France, 1996). That law passed 49/1
in the Senate and 90/0 in the House (10 members were absent). For many
legislators, hearing the moving personal story of what happened to a survivor was the first time they were able to understand what was at stake and
why they should pass such legislation. In the states that failed to pass legislation, survivors do not seem to have played a central role in lobbying or
testifying, though they were active in initiating the efforts.

The importance of survivor participation can be a problem in those
states that do not pass the legislation quickly. Many of the survivors suffer from burnout, and since the movement is so small, there is no ready
supply of replacements to keep the momentum going. On several occasions I was told by a survivor that she had been working for the legislation, which had so far failed, and, despite the obvious need for her
participation, she could no longer continue her efforts.

The influence of high-profile cases in initiating or pushing along efforts
to pass the legislation is also important. As we have seen, this is one of the
factors that distinguish successes from failures. As in the case of testimony
by survivors, these cases serve to anchor what is sometimes a murky issue.

SO, HOW WERE THE LAWS PASSED?

What is striking about the efforts to criminalize professional sexual misconduct is the absence of any distinguishable pattern. There is no single
"recipe" for success. In some states, the law was passed as the "ultimate
no-brainer," while in others, it took a concerted effort by various actors
over an extended period. However, even concerted efforts did not guarantee success; in some states (most notably Massachusetts) all the ingredients
that one would expect to lead to success have, instead, led to failure of suc-
cessive efforts. To add to the confusion, my research revealed that in some
successful states, related bills were later introduced and failed. In Arizona,
for example, a bill to extend the ban to the clergy failed, as did a bill in
South Dakota that would have required doctors to have a third person in
the examining room with patients to minimize the risk of doctor–patient
sex.

As we have seen, this case does not fit any of the models of the previous
research on when and how legislation is passed. Characteristics of the
state in which legislation was attempted seem in general to have less to do
with the eventual outcome of the efforts than other factors. Several factors
do, however, seem to have been associated with a successful outcome in

the case studied here, though there are insufficient cases for statistical analysis.

Ingredients in the Recipe for Success

1. An outrageous case, or preferably more than one, that receives wide media publicity, can trigger the belief that "something must be done." It is also helpful, though not necessary, if it is made clear in the media publicity that the existing remedies for dealing with such cases are inadequate or that the existence of a criminal statute might prevent survivors from filing costly civil cases. In a well-publicized case in Colorado, which was the subject of a *Firing Line* program, the victim made it clear that she considered a criminal remedy much more effective than the civil remedy she sought, as did a number of other victims she interviewed (Roberts-Henry, 1995). New Hampshire extended its law prohibiting sexual contact in a medical context to therapists after a court had concluded that a psychologist had engaged in "medical practice" under the existing statute (*State v. VonKlock* 433 A.2d 1299 N. H. 1981). That case pointed to the need for a legislative, rather than a judicial, remedy.

2. The support of powerful legislators (especially those on the relevant committee or, even better, its chair).

3. The support of institutions such as the state professional associations (especially the more prestigious ones, such as the psychiatric association and the medical association).

4. The absence of opposition from legislators and institutions (especially the clergy).

5. The presence of at least one articulate survivor able to personalize the issue and its importance.

6. Framing the issue as one in which consent of the patient is seen as irrelevant. Activist survivors play an important role in this framing process. In those states where the issue of consent became central, the bill was less likely to pass. In other cases, the bill was dropped because it was rewritten to limit its application only to nonconsensual sex, which adds nothing to current law (e.g., New Mexico on its first try and Michigan).

7. It also seems that the moment must be seized when the "policy window" is open, as Kingdon would argue (Kingdon, 1995). Rhode Island, which began its legislative effort fairly late, has seen interest wane after the bill failed twice to pass the House. As Senator Roney said: [P]olitically, the issue of therapist abuse is declining" (Roney, 1998).

8. The one characteristic of the state itself that seems to have been associated with legislative success is the political culture, as we saw earlier. States with more open polities, as defined by Elazar's classification of types of political culture, are more likely to have passed legislation.

In addition to these variables, idiosyncratic factors can play a role. For example, North Dakota, being adjacent to Minnesota, had the benefit of all the media interest in the Minnesota papers, which were read by people in North Dakota. In Texas, one survivor was very well connected politically and so was able to mobilize a great deal of support.

This research has shown that the passage of legislation is a rather unpredictable process, with different strategies working in some states and not in others, making theoretical prediction very difficult. Fortunately, activists and legislators seem to be willing to work for the passage of legislation about which they feel strongly even without a road map as to the best way to ensure the success of proposed legislation.

IMPLEMENTATION OF THE CRIMINAL LEGISLATION

Once legislation is passed, it is generally assumed that it will reduce and ideally eliminate whatever problem it was intended to address, in this case, sexual exploitation by professionals. For some, that can be measured by the increased salience of the issue caused by publicity surrounding the legislation. For others, actual criminal prosecutions represent a successful outcome. This section addresses both the small quantity of empirical data available to measure the implementation of these statutes as well as information about ways in which activists have framed the effects of the statutes.

Prosecutions under the Criminal Statutes

Obtaining data on criminal prosecutions under these statutes is particularly difficult. No national records are kept, as these crimes are not included in the Uniform Crime Report (UCR) statistics. Nor do states keep their own composite records of crimes not listed in the UCR. Surveying district attorneys for each county in a particular state is almost the only way to obtain figures for prosecutions under statutes such as these. Sometimes information can be obtained from well-connected professionals in the field or from state agencies, but this information can be unreliable and covers only limited areas.

Some information has been published on the implementation of the earliest statutes, in Wisconsin and Minnesota, but none about those states that passed their laws later. For this reason I conducted surveys of district attorneys in two states (Colorado and Maine) who had passed their statutes in 1988 and 1989, which would have been enough time to gather some information about their impact. The available data are described in the following section.

Wisconsin

In 1992 Andrew Kane (1995) conducted a survey of district attorneys in Wisconsin to determine how many cases they had prosecuted under the statute in the intervening nine years since the statute was passed. In response to his survey Kane found that a total of two cases were reported under the misdemeanor statute, which went into effect in 1983, and eight cases under the felony statute, which went into effect in 1986 (319). Kane also reports that by combining the information he obtained from the district attorneys with reports from newspapers and other sources, he has obtained information on a total of 30 convictions in the 10-year period between 1983 and the end of 1993. Of those 30 cases, however, 21 were charged under sexual assault statutes or other criminal statutes, rather than under the statute prohibiting sexual contact between a therapist and a patient (333).

Of the nine charged under the sexual exploitation statute, two were described as psychiatrists, one as a therapist (a female), two as clergymen, two as chemical dependency counselors, and two as counselors. Of those 21 charged under other statutes, clergymen featured most prominently (12). The rest were psychologists (two), social workers (two), one psychiatric resident, and four counselors (including one chemical dependency counselor, one school guidance counselor, and two unspecified) (329–32).

These figures seem to underline power (or lack thereof) in criminal prosecutions, in that among the professions subject to these laws, those with the least power in the helping profession hierarchy appear more likely to be prosecuted. Such an observation is, at this point, only conjecture, given the small numbers involved and the possibility that the apparent emphasis on lower-status professions may have occurred by chance. However, we see this trend duplicated in the empirical data I collected on Colorado, in which, for example, no psychiatrist has been charged under the statute. The incidence data do not indicate that a higher proportion of counselors or the clergy exploit their clients than do psychiatrists or psychologists; yet these latter professions feature relatively rarely in these prosecutions.

Minnesota

Some data are also available from Minnesota for the period from 1985 to 1992. I have combined the descriptions of the cases prosecuted under the Minnesota statute provided by Schoener with that obtained from the Minnesota Board of Medical Practice until 1992 (Schoener, 1989d: 553–60; Minnesota Board of Medical Examiners, 1992). These two sources yield a total of 16 cases. Of those prosecutions, 12 resulted in conviction, and 1 was pending at the time the data were gathered. The professions prosecuted were as follows: psychologists (five), clergy (four), chemical dependency counselors (three), psychiatric resident (one), social worker (female—one), "psychic guide" (one), and profession unknown (one). While more psychologists were prosecuted here than in Wisconsin, psychiatrists are noticeable by their absence, a further indication that prosecutions may be disproportionately brought against less powerful professions. Recent information from the Minnesota Board of Medical Practice indicates that only one physician has been convicted under the statute in the last four years (Erickson, 1998). According to Gary Schoener (19 May 1998) of the Walk-In Counselling Center, there have been about 20 cases to date.

Colorado and Maine

In 1995 I sent surveys to district attorneys in Colorado and Maine in an effort to add to the data described earlier about the implementation of these statutes. Now that there is a critical mass of statutes, one ought to be better able to determine their overall impact, especially as the subject has been getting more attention recently. Colorado and Maine were selected because, after Minnesota and Wisconsin, they passed their statutes early, in 1988 and 1989. Table 7.3 shows the results for Colorado, and Table 7.4, for Maine.

The tables for Colorado and Maine show that these statutes are used very rarely. In Maine only one case was prosecuted. In Colorado a total of 27 professionals were charged under the statute in the five years since it

Table 7.3
Colorado Survey Results: Prosecutions for Sexual Assault on a Client by a Psychotherapist

The response rate was 86% (19 of 22). Not everyone answered every question, so the number of respondents was often less than 19 for any particular question.

1) Have you prosecuted any psychotherapists, clergy, physicians, etc. under the state felony or misdemeanor statute (s. 18-3-405.5) in the period since the statute was passed in 1989?

YES: 7	NO: 11	NO RESPONSE: 1

2 a) If yes, how many felony cases of aggravated sexual assault (s. 18-3-405.5 (1))?

	1.	2.	Total
1990	2		2
1991	1	1	3
1992	3		3
1993	2	1	4
1994	1		1
Year unspecified			1
TOTAL			14

2 b) How many misdemeanor cases of sexual assault (18-3-405.5)?

	1.	2.	Total
1990		1	2
1991		1	2
1992	1	1	2
1993		1	2
1994		1	2
TOTAL			13

(Continued)

Table 7.3
(Continued)

3) For each of the following professional affiliations, please write in the total number of cases prosecuted for each of the following years.

	1990	1991	1992	1993	1994	Total
Psychologist	1	1	1		1	4
Psychiatrist						
Physician	1	1	2	2		6
Clergy *	1	2	1	1		6
Massage Therapist					1	1
Chiropractor					1	1
Dentist					1	1
TOTAL						20

*One year unspecified

4) Please indicate the total number of male and female defendants for each of the following years:

	1990	1991	1992	1993	1994	Total
Male	3	6	6	6	2	23
Female					1	1

5) For each of the following categories, please indicate the total number reported to your office for each of the following years:

	1990	1991	1992	1993	1994	Total
Victim	2	3	4	3	2	14
Other therapist	1	1	1			3

6) For each of the following disposition categories, please indicate the total number of cases handled for each of the following years:

	1990	1991	1992	1993	1994	Total
Charges dropped		1	2	2	1	6
Acquitted			1	1	1	3
Convicted	3	5	5	3	3	19

7) Of those cases resulting in conviction, what were the sentences for each of the following years?

	1990	1991	1992	1993	1994	Total
Probation	3	2	2	1		8
Fine		2				2
Imprisonment		2	2	1		5
Other (public service no contact)	1	1	1	1	1	5

8) Do you believe that the criminalization of sexual misconduct by psychotherapists has had a positive impact on the incidence of that misconduct?

YES: 7 NO: 1 NOT ENOUGH INFORMATION: 3

(In addition, one massage therapist was reported but not charged in the 20th District because the job description did not fit into the definition of therapist. However, a massage therapist was prosecuted in another district.)

was passed; 19 were convicted. Jorgenson, Randles, and Strasburger (1991: 674) argue that at least some of the statutes, as in Maine, are set up in such a way as to make successful prosecution very difficult by defining terms, such as "therapy," very narrowly. The results of the Maine survey seem to bear out this view. The Colorado statute, however, which uses more broadly defined terms, is nevertheless used infrequently. The New Mexico

The Wages of Seeking Help

Table 7.4
Maine Survey Results: Prosecutions for Sexual Assault on a Client by a Therapist

The response rate was 63% (five out of eight districts responded).	

1) Have you prosecuted any psychiatrists, psychologists, or social workers under the state criminal statute (ME. REV. STAT. ANN. tit. 17-A., s.253(2)(I)) in the period since the statute was passed in 1989?

   YES: 1   NO: 4

2) If yes, how many cases of gross sexual assault?

   2 (same person, no year specified)

3) For each of the following professional affiliations, please write in the total number of cases prosecuted for each of the following years.

	1990	1991	1992	1993	1994	Unknown
Psychologist						
Psychiatrist						
Social Worker *						2
TOTAL						

   * Same person

4) Please indicate the total number of male and female defendants for each of the following years:

	1990	1991	1992	1993	1994	Unknown
Male						1
Female						

5) For each of the following categories, please indicate the total number reported to your office for each of the following years:

   No Response

6) For each of the following disposition categories, please indicate the total number of cases handled for each of the following years:

	1990	1991	1992	1993	1994	Unknown
Convicted						1
Convicted of Other Charges						1

7) Of those cases resulting in conviction, what were the sentences for each of the following years?

	1990	1991	1992	1993	1994	Unknown
Fine						1

8) Do you believe that the criminalization of sexual misconduct by therapists has had a positive impact on the incidence of that misconduct?

   YES: 1   ·   NO: NOT ENOUGH INFORMATION: 1

statute is also more broadly defined and had not been used at all by 1995 but has been used at least twice since (Noel, 1998).

General Effects: Publicity and Deterrence

Kane (1995) argues that these statutes serve both a punitive and a deterrent purpose. Even though the statutes do not appear to serve the purpose of punishment very well, as the results of the various surveys show, they might be serving a deterrent purpose. Such a claim is, however, very difficult to substantiate. Eighty-seven percent of Kane's district attorney respondents said that they believed that criminalization of professional sexual misconduct has had a positive impact on the incidence of this behavior (325). My district attorney respondents were less convinced (37 percent in Colorado; 20 percent in Maine).

Kane also asked a sample of psychologists in Wisconsin about the deterrent effect of the criminalization of professional sexual contact. Seventy-nine percent of them said that the statute had had a positive impact on incidence. It should be noted, however, that 28 percent of the psychologist respondents indicated that the criminal statute had a negative effect on their practice (such as increased anxiety or stress, worry about frivolous accusations). The legislation is evidently not without negative consequences for the practitioner.

Proving deterrence is particularly difficult in this case. Pope and Vasquez (1991: 102) argue, on the basis of incidence studies over a period of time, that there has been a "fairly consistent decrease in the rate" of involvement. They speculate that the decline could be genuine and "caused by such factors as the increasing criminalization of this behavior" as well as several other factors. They also admit, however, that the decline could represent "less candid reporting." Schoener (1991) argues that incidence studies cannot be used to indicate a decline in the rate, because of their many limitations as well as differences among them that prevent comparison. Schoener (19 May 1998) does believe that the incidence and prevalence have "dropped dramatically" in Minnesota but attributes the drop to a number of factors rather than just the legislation. He cites as one piece of evidence the fact that the therapist who has been conducting groups for victims of professional sexual exploitation was unable this year to get enough people for the group, for the first time in 20 years. He believes that the combination of Minnesota's entire package of measures has reduced the problem. He points to the civil statute (which he argues has "nailed more people than the criminal statute"), mandatory reporting, extensive public hearings, public education and professional training.

In any assessment of the deterrent value of legislation, including Kane's survey of psychologists discussed earlier, it is implicit that the targets actually know about the existence of the legislation. My experience with interviewing professionals for this research makes me question that this is, indeed, the case. A remarkable number of those I interviewed whose names had been given to me as informants knowledgeable about the statutes did not know of their existence, including people in central positions in the relevant professional organizations. Many people confused the criminal statutes with the licensing statutes or were simply unaware that such a statute had been passed.

In Texas a recent study of social workers showed that many of them were not familiar with the provisions of the legislation (Sloan et al., 1998). A sample of 450 social workers in Texas were given a questionnaire that included eight questions on various aspects of the legislation on sexual exploitation by psychotherapists. Half of the respondents answered half of the questions correctly. No respondent was able to answer all the questions correctly, and seven respondents answered none correctly.

Further support for an argument that neither professionals nor the public is aware of the passage of these laws comes from the material about media publicity of the legislative efforts described in the first part of this chapter. As reported earlier (Sloan et al., 1998), in most cases there was very little media publicity about the statutes. The trigger cases, which made more exciting copy for newspapers, were more likely to be reported, but the legislation itself was not extensively publicized. In at least one case (Connecticut), this was purposeful behavior on the part of those seeking the legislation, on the premise that the lower the profile of the bill, the less likely opposition would mobilize. While this was apparently a successful strategy in that state, it did not serve to publicize the existence of the law once it was passed.

To provide more empirical material of the extent to which professionals are informed about the criminal statute, I surveyed all the state psychological associations in states that had passed legislation. One obvious place to inform professionals about the new legislation would be through the association newsletter, so I asked whether there had been any information in the newsletter when the statute had been passed or since. A number of the executive directors did not themselves know of the legislation to which I was referring, but I was able to get information in most cases about the publicity of the statutes. Not surprisingly, Minnesota was the state with the most publicity, most notably in a series of articles written by Gary Schoener over the years. Wisconsin, Colorado, and California also had some publicity. The rest of the states either did not mention the legislation at all in their newsletters or had a paragraph at the time it was passed, generally as part of a description of other relevant legislation (e.g., Morris and Perrin, 1994).

A few states have made some efforts to inform patients of their rights in therapy, which include their options if they have been exploited, one of which is to file a criminal complaint with the police in the states with criminal legislation. Without the impetus from potential complainants, it is extremely unlikely that the police would prosecute. They have "more important" things to do with their resources. While it is possible for complaints to be initiated by therapists, and in a few states they are *required* to report any suspected cases, therapists are reluctant to do so for a variety of reasons. The information in Table 7.3 for Colorado showed that only three of the cases were reported by a therapist. In any event, the reporting requirements are to the licensing authorities and not to the police. There appears to be very little exchange of such information between the licensing authorities and the police to facilitate prosecution by the criminal justice authorities.

CONCLUSION

We have seen in this chapter the variety of ways in which the legislation to criminalize therapist–patient sex has been passed and some of the forces that seem to increase the likelihood that efforts to pass legislation will be successful. The issue of whether these statutes "work" in solving or reducing the problem is much more difficult to assess. I have attempted to show that the criminal statutes do not appear to be used very much. Clearly, even if the lowest-incidence figures are used, there is much more therapist–patient sex taking place than is the subject of criminal charges. It is also clear that even among the people for whom this is an important issue, especially professionals, the level of awareness is very low. The deterrent value of legislation clearly comes from a recognition of the criminality of such behavior, which is not possible if a potential offender is unaware of the existence of the criminal statute.

That is not to say, however, that the legislation has had no effect at all on the problem. But it appears that its effect is likely to be much greater when it is one prong of a multipronged attack on the problem, including civil statutes and reporting laws, discussed in Chapter 6, and the strengthening of licensing requirements, discussed in Chapter 8. There is, however, relatively little evidence that those involved in the training of professionals have done much to address this issue (Schoener, 1997). Nor is there much evidence of public awareness of the problem. If there is to be genuine change in this area, passing a law by itself is insufficient. It has to be implemented by the criminal justice authorities, and it also has to be a part of a package of legal reform, education, and information before there will be real change.

NOTE

1. Bisbing et al.'s (1999) list is more extensive than mine, as they also include statutes that are worded much more broadly. For example, they include Ohio's statute, which includes under sexual battery, situations of coercion or inability to appraise the nature of the act (Ohio Rev. Code Ann, ss 2907.03[2]). They also include Rhode Island, where, I have been told, the legislation has twice passed the Senate but has not passed the House (John Roney, 1998). The statutes I include are those that directly address the issue of therapist–patient sex.

— 8 —

REGULATION

I had no idea how awful this thing was going to be. These guys [on the committee] were just awful. I felt I was on trial. I think it was more humiliating than the abuse. They asked me all kinds of questions about my sexual history. . . . they kept asking the same questions over and over . . . every little detail, and they asked me all these irrelevant questions. . . . It was all designed to get me to back out.
—A victim exploited as a teenager, about her complaint before the State Ethics Committee

INTRODUCTION

This chapter addresses the regulation of professional sexual misconduct by the professional associations and licensing boards. For the most part, it focuses on regulation of professions other than the clergy, as each religious denomination has its own policies and procedures, about which very little information is available. It also does not address lawyer sexual misconduct, for, as we have seen, very few states have banned attorney–client sexual conduct. Claims of such behavior to disciplinary authorities are likely to be dismissed without any investigation (Langford, 1995). As this issue has begun to receive more attention, some changes in regulation and statutes have been made. Those changes have themselves succeeded in increasing the attention paid to the issues but do not appear to have had much effect on the rate of prosecution of the misbehavior. Nor do they appear to have reduced the trauma described by survivor after survivor, most of whom echo the sentiment of the victim quoted at the beginning of the chapter. In addition, professionals who have been the subject of complaints have similar objections to the process. In this chapter, I argue that the reason little has changed is that agencies are caught in the middle of a number of conflicting pressures that make it impossible for them to satisfy their various constituents.

Those involved in regulation argue that they have begun to pay more attention to the problem and are handling it with appropriate seriousness. Victims continue to argue that they are still treated so badly that some choose not to take their complaints before regulatory agencies. Social movement activists support the contention of the victims that very little has changed. Professionals who have been charged with misconduct see the regulatory system as nothing less than a witch-hunt designed to hound some of those who are not part of the mainstream professional power structure.

PROFESSIONAL REGULATION: GENERAL ISSUES

As we saw in Chapter 3, a victim has a number of avenues for redress when she first perceives that she has been harmed. Schoener et al. (1989), in their classic work on professional sexual misconduct, provide what they call a "Wheel of Options," which offers no fewer than 12 different choices available to the victim, ranging from doing nothing, to contacting her ex-counselor, to more official options (308). All of the options are not available to every victim; for example, only those exploited by a member of the clergy can notify the church hierarchy, and criminal complaints are available only in some states. This chapter deals with two of the most widely available options: a licensure complaint and a complaint to the ethics committee of the appropriate professional association. Through these two mechanisms, especially the former, most professions are controlled. The major "helping" professions are, for the most part, required to be licensed (though, as we have seen in Chapter 6, it is possible to be a "therapist" without being licensed), and many professionals belong to their professional association.

Sociologists have devoted attention to understanding the nature of the professions and the increase both in their number and in their power (e.g., Dingwall and Lewis, 1983; Johnson, 1972; Brint, 1994). They define a professional in a variety of ways, one of which is the degree of autonomy they maintain over their work. One of the ways they protect this autonomy is through the mechanism of self-regulation (Constantinides, 1991). The justification for this self-regulation is found in the argument that only those trained in the profession are in a position to evaluate appropriately the professional qualifications and actions of their colleagues.

According to Constantinides (1991: 1333), this self-regulation has three components: "1) control of recruitment and certification; 2) creation of an ethics code; and 3) a professional review mechanism." The second and third components of professional self-regulation concern us here. In general, professions that are involved in counseling or therapy have some form of specific ethics rule that outlaws sexual behavior between professional and patient or client. For example, the Code of Ethics of the National

Association of Social Workers states: "The social worker should not under any circumstances engage in sexual activities with clients" (*NASW Code of Ethics*, 1993: 5). The most notable exception is the legal profession, which has a prohibition only in a very few states (Jorgenson, 1995a).

The professional review mechanism is the process mentioned earlier for handling the complaints about sexual misconduct from patients and clients as well as (at least in theory) other professionals. In those professions that have a specific rule against sexual involvement with a patient or a client, the issue is, in fact, not determining whether the behavior can be considered appropriate professional practice but, rather, credibility: did the events complained of actually happen? Once the sexual behavior is established, the question becomes not whether some action should take place but what action (Lehr, 1994). Thus, in this context at least, the profession itself has no special ability to determine the answer to this question. In fact, such expertise resides in the legal system. Lawyers and judges are constantly involved in issues of credibility.

How well this system works in practice is the subject of periodic debate, both in general and in relation to particular professions (e.g., Dolan and Urban, 1983; Bayles, 1986; Clark, 1981). While there have been proposals for radical change in the regulatory mechanism, the system remains basically intact. There has been some movement to have lay representation on licensing boards, but, for the most part, this has been no more than token representation and not very effective (Dolan and Urban, 1983). Perhaps the most significant change that has taken place is a dramatic increase in the number of occupations that define themselves as professions and claim the corresponding privilege of self-regulation (Bayles, 1986).

As we have seen, it is very difficult to determine how well the system of self-regulation is working to prevent and punish sexual misconduct. Professional regulation takes place in such a variety of contexts that it is particularly difficult to determine what is going on. Each profession has its own national organization (and such organizations vary in the extent to which they involve themselves in individual complaints), as well as state and local organizations with their own practices and procedures for handling ethics complaints. In addition, each state has a licensing authority for a varying number of professions, again with its own practices and procedures, including considerable discretion as well as variation in the scope of its power (Bisbing et al., 1995: 859).

From the consumer's point of view, even figuring out to whom and how to lodge a complaint is a major accomplishment. One could be forgiven for wondering whether this is the result of an ambivalence about the process on the part of those involved in professional regulation. Whatever the reason, the result is a low rate of complaints compared to the evidence about the incidence of professional sexual misconduct. Some states have undertaken major efforts to make this information available to the public (e.g., Minnesota and Maryland), but most have done very little. The Maryland task force report states that "it has been found that only a minority of cases are actually reported" ("Sexual Exploitation," 1996: 1). The Report of the Committee on Physician Sexual Misconduct in Ontario reported that of the 208 callers to the toll-free line who complained of having been sexually exploited by a physician, only 23 actually reported the incident to the College of Physicians and Surgeons responsible for licensing and regulation (*Crossing the Boundaries*, 1992: 65). In a Rhode Island study, only one sexual misconduct case was reported to the Board of Examiners in Psychology during a three-year period, although a survey among subsequent therapists reported at least 37 incidents by psychologists during the same period (Parsons and Wincze, 1995). This figure is also lower than the total number of incidents since many victims do not return to therapy. Vinson's (1987) study in California showed that lack of knowledge rather than lack of motivation prevented women from filing complaints about professional sexual misconduct. Bouhoutsos et al.'s (1983) study of psychologists who treated patients sexually exploited by previous therapists indicated that only 52 percent of 559 victims knew that their therapist's behavior was unethical or illegal, only 4 percent took legal action, 3 percent filed professional complaints, and 3 percent notified the state licensing board. Low reporting rates get even lower when one looks at the outcome of those reports. The Report of the Public Citizen Health Research Group compared the rate of discipline with the incidence rate, as shown in the various surveys of the medical profession over the last 25 years (Dehlendorf and Wolfe, 1997: 21–22). Using the data from 1994, the year of the highest rate of discipline (0.023 percent), they argue that, assuming a physician is at risk for discipline for, at most, 50 years, the greatest chance that a physician could be disciplined for a sex-related offense in his lifetime is 1.2 percent. By contrast, the prevalence studies point to a rate of offending of between 3.5 percent and 15 percent, which suggests that 66 percent to 91 percent of physicians who commit sex-related offenses will never be disciplined. Even allowing for several limitations in these calculations, as Dehlendorf and Wolfe do, these figures point to a very low rate of action by regulatory authorities in response to the problem.

As far as can be determined from the little available information, most of the complaints that are filed come from the victims themselves, rather than from fellow professionals, even though professional self-regulation is intended to rely on peer review to identify and evaluate behavior (see *Crossing the Boundaries*, 1992, Appendix A: 29; Bisbing et al., 1995: 865). Despite the underlying philosophy of peer evaluation, most professionals have a very difficult time blowing the whistle on their colleagues. They appear to have even more difficulty denying them their livelihoods by removing a license after a professional has been found to have behaved unprofessionally, as illustrated by the extremely low rate of license revocation in the available data (e.g., Lehr, 1994; *Task Force*, 1991: 21). This is true both at an individual level and at an institutional level. One study revealed that medical societies rarely report physicians to the state licensing officials. In six years and 6,378 reports, only 106 came from medical societies ("Malpractice Crisis," 1986).

Professionals possess significant power in our society (Bayles, 1986; Friedson, 1986). Bayles argues that the primary source of professional power is the claim to expertise, a claim he believes is exaggerated (31–32). In the context of professional sexual misconduct, this professional power is closely connected to gender, which increases the power of the professional vis-à-vis the complainant. For Quadrio (1994), the sexual misconduct is itself "an expression of the male therapist's need to assert power and dominance over his female patients" (193).

The social roles of the person in need of help and the person administering that help exacerbate the power imbalance, especially when the patient or client is female. In fact, the relationship of the fatherly professional responding to the needs of the childlike patient or client is the archetypical patriarchal relationship. These social roles color the adjudication of complaints. As long as those hearing them represent the father and those complaining represent the child (usually female), the former is far more likely to be believed than the latter. Many victims complain that the system is stacked in favor of the doctors: "The present system . . . is seen by victims as a system that is run by doctors, that is controlled by doctors, and which exists for doctors" (*Task Force*, 1991: 84). They describe the treatment they received during the complaint process as including hostility, not being believed, and not being kept informed of what is happening (*Task Force*, 1991: 87). For some victims, it all looks like a professional "club," with the victim the only person outside it (Bisbing et al., 1995: 884). One victim wrote that "a report to the board makes me an enemy of their community—their 'in-group'" (K. B., 1999). "The Board really gives people a hard time; they are protecting him, scared of being sued," Janie told me (Janie, 1999). Most victims agree that the process is a negative one; other observers show that it is also badly managed. In his study of the Massachusetts system of professional regulation, Lehr (1994) concludes that the system is "a regulatory effort beset by delays, poor record-keeping and a lack of real clout" (1). The Task Force on Sexual Abuse of patients in Ontario reported that "with two exceptions, the complainants we met with had found the process to be daunting, devaluing, and retraumatizing. Most described it as being as abusive and harmful to them as the original abuse" (*Task Force*, 1991: 87). One complainant even described the letter sent to her by the board as "powerfully discouraging, even intimidating" (K. B., 1999). My research, for the most part, supports this view, though more recently it appears that some boards are being more supportive. "I have to say that everyone throughout the process was very sensitive to my feelings and attempted to put me at ease. I never felt ridiculed or put down (only by my former psychiatrist)," Linda told me (Linda, 1999).

METHODS OF CONTROL OF SEXUAL MISCONDUCT

Licensing Boards

Introduction

If a victim is able to make her way through the tangle of licensing boards and is willing to risk being treated badly, she has a real incentive to file a complaint against her perpetrator with his licensing board, which has the power to punish the professional for his misconduct, a punishment up to and including the revocation of his license to practice his profession. Once victims realize how they have been harmed by the professional sexual misconduct, they express concern that the professional will continue to exploit others in the same way with equally damaging results. As one victim said: "I decided to file a licensing board complaint because I didn't want another victim on my conscience. I did a very long and intensive soul searching about what the pros and cons were regarding exposing HIM and ultimately decided the best courses of action were with the Social Work Licensing Board and the civil suit (both of these having the most power and the least revictimizing)" (Nancy, 1999).

While the potential for revocation is the main advantage of a licensing board complaint for the victim, there are also other advantages. Plaut and Foster (1986) list a number of the advantages of the process, including the fact that the decisions of boards are rarely overturned and that statutes of limitations, which are so problematic in civil suits, do not usually apply. Illinois, with its one-year limitation, is an exception to the general rule, though the case can be reopened if the professional association takes action. In a licensing complaint one does not need a lawyer, as one does in a civil suit. A successful outcome from a licensing board can help significantly in the civil claim and vice versa, so some victims do have lawyers in complaints to the board, though they have no official role.

For many victims, however, these advantages may not actually exist, or they may be outweighed by disadvantages. For example, revocation is rarely the outcome of the complaint procedure; more often, a lesser punishment is negotiated. Most boards are very reluctant, except in what they see as the most egregious cases in which rehabilitation seems impossible, to deny a fellow professional his livelihood. They may try to persuade the professional to surrender his license, which saves the time, expense, and trauma to the victim but denies those victims who want "a day in court" the sense of vindication that may come from testifying. "Voluntary" surrender has risks of its own; one therapist was told to turn in his license under the emergency provisions because of a suicide attempt and later claimed that he had surrendered his license under duress. A variety of other plea bargains are also common, which have the same impact on the victim. Surrender seems to be more frequent than revocation, though it is difficult to determine this, as many boards combine those figures into one category, "loss of license." Data collected by the Federation of Medical Boards of the United States indicate that in 1992 (the latest year for which figures are broken down in this way), of 42 boards reporting, 2 physicians had their licenses denied, while 23 surrendered them (Winn, 1993). These data are supported by the Dehlendorf and Wolfe (1997) report, which indicates that the severity of discipline remains low, and in fact, the percentage of orders that included a revocation or surrender of license decreased from 47.2 percent to 36.2 percent between 1989 and 1994, the period of the study (8). Also, boards often use orders of suspension rather than revocation. This is partly because it is possible for a therapist who has had his license revoked to practice as an unlicensed therapist beyond the control of the board. Using suspension with conditions gives the board more control over the therapist and is also related to the belief that sex-related offending is a relatively easily cured problem.

Boards are also concerned that a revocation is likely to be appealed to the courts, adding to their expense and the time it takes to resolve the case. For these reasons, some states virtually never revoke the license of a professional against whom a complaint has been made. For example, in Colorado, eight psychologists were charged with "sexual intimacies," or "sex with patient," between 1987 and 1994. None of them had their licenses revoked. The only psychologist who had his license revoked was charged with sexual harassment rather than sexual behavior with a patient (Schmitt, 1995). In my own research, I found that the rate of revocation of physicians charged with sexual misconduct with their patients varied considerably from state to state, ranging from 1 revocation in Iowa over a five-year period to 69 in New York.

In many cases, rather than being able to use the outcome of the complaint process in the civil suit, boards put their process on hold, pending the outcome of the lawsuit. "I was later informed by others that the Board wouldn't finish my case until the lawsuit was over because their decisions could prejudice either him or me in the lawsuit. . . . if they had sanctioned him, then we could have used that at trial and then it may have prejudiced the jury and not given him a fair trial—or vice versa," Paula told me (Paula, 1999). During that period, as during the board investigation of the complaint (which also can take months or years), the professional continues to practice, much to the outrage of many victims.

How the Process Works

The procedures for filing a complaint vary considerably among boards (for details, see Bisbing et al., 1995: 862–64). The complaint usually has to be in writing, which itself is seen as a barrier to reporting by some victims, especially those who are unsophisticated in the ways of the law and the need for due process. More than one of the victims I interviewed initially made inquiries of the board anonymously. Doubtless, many victims proceed no further than that. One victim felt discouraged by the response to the anonymous phone call to the board to find out her rights if she reported. "They were impatient, abrupt, and said several times they couldn't tell me unless I first told them who and what I was reporting" (K. B., 1999). Once a complaint has been made, the board conducts its own inquiry in order to decide whether there is enough evidence to proceed further. If that decision is affirmative, the board begins a formal investigation, at which time the case becomes a matter of public record. Several of the victims I interviewed, however, say that, in fact, the information is not really public at this time. One victim from Arizona told me that the board was supposed to post the information on its Web site but has not done so. Another said that "it seems like the results of this case have been so hush-hush." The data collection phase is followed by a hearing at which the victim usually must confront her perpetrator and present testimony of her complaint. These hearings can be extensive; the longest one I heard about was scheduled in two parts, three days at one time and then five days three months later. The final decision is made sometime after the hearing and may involve complex negotiations about the terms of the punishment. Judicial review is also available for the professional to appeal the decision. The ruling of an administrative law judge may or may not be binding on the board. In California the Board of Psychologists frequently does not accept the ruling of the administrative judge who reviews the case (*PAN meeting*, 1996).

While the preceding description provides the bare outline of the process, it does not reflect the many different approaches to regulation in the many boards involved (Schoener, 1994). Some hearings are open, while others are closed. Victims generally prefer open hearings, which make them feel less excluded. The investigators of the case may vary from board to board. Some places use Federal Bureau of Investigation (FBI) agents who have training in investigation, though not in health cases. Others use nurses or other professionals as investigators who do know health cases but may not know what to look for. Victims I interviewed had mixed reactions to the people who investigated their complaints. "It took three months to get to talk to my investigator at my urging. The investigator didn't give me much information, nor did he ask me many questions to confirm or deny what my therapist used as a defense. It took several months more to learn what was going on," one victim told me. Another complained of the extensive turnover in investigators during the investigation of her complaint. On the more positive side, one victim said her investigator was wonderful. "It was like telling your grandmother what had happened."

States vary in who hears the case. Members of the board may hear the case, or there may be a legal examiner. This can be an administrative law judge who may or may not know about professional sexual exploitation or relevant mental health issues. Boards also vary in who tries the case. In Canada private lawyers are hired for the purpose, while in the United States assistant attorneys general are used, which is cheaper, though there are problems with them. These cases may not be a very high priority or an area of expertise for them. Boards are notoriously underfunded, which is one of the reasons they have such a large backlog of cases.

The Empirical Data

No national study of the actions of regulatory boards exists in complaints of professional sexual misconduct. Public Citizen Health Research Group has published one study of the medical profession, and the Federation of State Medical Boards of the United States occasionally extracts the data on sexual misconduct of physicians from the material sent to them by individual state boards. When I began the research for this chapter, I attempted to undertake a national survey of data obtained from state professional associations and licensing boards responsible for the control of professional sexual misconduct to determine how well the system is working. This proved impossible because precise, comparable data could not be obtained. Statistics are not kept in ways that make comparison possible; standards vary; and changes have taken place at different times in different states in the way data are kept, making even within-state comparison over time impossible. Some boards recently added a separate category for sexual misconduct, while others still have no special category but use such labels as dual relationships. Others have more than one label, for example, sexual intimacies and sexual improprieties. Likewise, states label their actions differently; a suspension in one state may not mean the same thing as a suspension in another. In addition, there are a number of different licensing authorities in each state that license a different, but extensive, list of professionals. Although much of this information is supposed to be part of the public record, some of the licensing boards and professional associations were extremely reluctant to provide me with data.

It is also apparent that, in some cases, the data provided by the boards are inaccurate. When the *Boston Globe* did its investigative reporting about medical regulation in Massachusetts in 1994, reporters examined the files themselves and found a number of cases that the board did not include in the figures it publicized (Lehr, 1994). The *Globe* reported that "(t)wo weeks after a recent request for sex abuse cases, the board produced the names of 23 psychiatrists. Missing were 16 psychiatrists whom the board had investigated for sexual misconduct that the *Globe* learned about from news clips and interviewing attorneys and victims" (Lehr, 1994: 14). Boards also vary in whether they report pending cases or not, thereby adding to the confusion. Another problem appears to be inaccuracies in classification of cases as sexual misconduct. The Florida Department of Business and Professional Regulation provided me with the final orders of several cases it had in 1994. One of them was the case of a nurse who, as part of a pattern of erratic behavior, also accused physicians of sexual misconduct and of running a covert prostitution and slavery ring (*Department of Business and Professional Regulation v. Price*, 1994). Clearly, her license was revoked, not for her sexual misconduct but for her psychological problems. Nevertheless, it was included in the data as a case of professional sexual misconduct.

Given this range of methodological difficulties, it is no wonder that there have been so few studies of the actions of licensing boards. I finally gave up on efforts to obtain national data in favor of a piecemeal approach of obtaining information from those few, mostly local studies that do exist and interviews with those involved in the system.

Based on this information, two general conclusions can be drawn. First, there has definitely been an overall increase in the number of claims filed and an increase in the number of cases on which boards have taken action. My research, while not providing much usable data, did point clearly to the conclusion that both complaints and actions had increased (Bohmer, 1995b). The report of the Federation of State Medical Boards on sexual misconduct by physicians was conducted on data from 1990 to 1992 that reviewed all cases of professional sexual misconduct reported by the state boards (Winn, 1993). It found 84 reported cases on which action had been taken in 1990, 101 in 1991, and 132 in 1992 (89). A later report shows some increase in cases on which actions were taken: 237 in 1993, 252 in 1995, and 232 in 1996 (News Release, 1997, Chart 6). Data were also provided of the ratio of complaints to actions taken, though only for the year 1992, based on responses from 42 boards. That year, there were 393 complaints, of which 81 were dismissed, 18 were settled by agreement, 37 resulted in action, and 257 were currently under investigation (Winn, 1993: 91). Dehlendorf and Wolfe (1997) report on data from 1989 to 1994 and show that over that period, the number of disciplinary orders for sex-related offenses increased from 47 to 162 (6–7).

Second, there is great variation among the different boards about how aggressively they pursue complaints of professional sexual misconduct, which may parallel their policy generally, or may only apply in the case of complaints of sexual misconduct. This finding, which I found in my own research, was supported by the other commentators. A 1995 memorandum from the Florida Agency for Health Care Administration proudly proclaimed that "last year, the Board of Medicine was nationally recognized as one of the most active regulatory medical boards [second only to California] in the country" ("State of Florida," 1995: 1). However, the Federation of State Medical Boards reports that in 1996 Florida had a total of 265 actions in a population of approximately 39,000 physicians, while

Arizona had 234 actions with only 13,576 physicians, and Texas had 243 actions in a population of 45,581 physicians. There has been very little speculation as to why there is so much variation among states. It may have to do with a number of factors, ranging from the amount of money provided by the state for investigation of complaints, to public pressure, to the way the system is administered. As we have seen, professional sexual misconduct has received some publicity over the last decade, which is not likely to have gone unnoticed by regulatory agencies. The Federation of State Medical Boards reported that the proportion of sexual misconduct actions to all actions doubled between 1990 and 1995 from 2.6 percent to 5.3 percent (News Release, 1997, Chart 2).

A Typical Case

K describes a story that is typical of the victims who complain of sexual misconduct to licensing authorities. She was diagnosed as having bipolar disorder by an internist, who referred her to a licensed professional counselor (LPC). Unknown to K, the LPC was treating the internist for sexual addiction, which did not prevent her from suggesting that K and her internist should meet for lunch to deal with her "intimacy problem." The lunch meetings soon developed into a sexual relationship. Later, K, who was very unstable, began to see a competent psychiatrist, who told the medical board of the behavior of the internist, as she was obligated to do. The board just put the information in the file and took no action. K herself complained to the board when her health improved. When the board found out that she was suing her internist in civil court, it put her complaint on hold until the outcome of that suit. "I was devastated that the doctor was still practicing." It was not until three years after the complaint that the board finally had a hearing. By this time, K had moved away and was summoned back at her own expense to testify. "They gave me ten days notice; I had said 'please give me notice,' but they didn't, so I had to pay $1000 to fly back. The hearing was very intimidating. They were all men, sitting on a podium, they made no eye contact with me. The physician was in the room staring at me. That made me very uncomfortable. He had a barrage of attorneys with him. I had no lawyer with me, it was too expensive. I had legal documents to back it up. After I finished my story they said the doctor wanted to say something. I was totally unprepared for that. Initially, he denied it, I was a liar, had fabricated it all. He spewed twelve step recovery jargon, so sorry he had done this. Then I had to leave, but he got to stay. I felt they could say anything about me and I couldn't defend myself." The board decided to revoke his license but to stay the revocation and put him on five years' probation. "I was told by my lawyer that this was the best option. He would have appealed the revocation, which would have taken another couple of years, without monitoring. They felt for the public safety, it was a better option."

K's experience with the Licensed Professional Counseling Board, to which she complained about the counselor who referred her to the internist, knowing he had a sexual addiction, was even less satisfactory. The board investigated the case over an extended period. K flew back at her own expense to that hearing also. Several months after the hearing, she received a letter saying that it acknowledged that the LPC had violated the code of ethics, though it violated its own procedures by failing to order one of the three stated options in such a case (revocation, reprimand, or probation). Instead, it required the counselor to take an ethics course at a local college and placed in her record information about the board decision.

Like many victims, K's experience was better in her civil suit. Both her case against the internist and her case against the LPC were ultimately settled for a substantial amount out of court. However, several issues remain troubling to her. First, the internist had such support in the community that she felt isolated and punished, and she and her family had to move away from the area. She lost friendships as a result of the case. "Wives of physicians in town told me they couldn't be seen with me." Second, the internist seems to have been very successful in convincing the community that he has made amends. There were several letters in the local paper, one saying that "there is always a woman out there, trying to bring powerful men down." All the letters were in support of the physician, generally saying what a wonderful person he was, a sentiment echoed by the paid ad he placed in the same paper.

Sources of Conflict: Tikvah's Story

It has become received wisdom in this field that victims generally have a bad experience when they complain to licensing boards. After interviewing many victims, I have come to the conclusion that inherent conflicts in the process make it extremely likely that the process will be perceived as negative by the complainant. The following case illustrates why this is often so.

Some victims are so wounded that it is hard to imagine any circumstances in which they would be happy with the outcome of the regulatory board. Take Tikvah, for example. She was exploited over a period of several years by a physician who was treating her for a serious medical condition. He had sex with her in his office and also saw her outside of his office, where he also medicated her, resulting in her having what she described as "steroid psychosis." He attempted to date her, had sex with her in her home (which was seen by her son), and also was sexually intimate with her when she was in the hospital. She says that both his partners and staff at the hospital knew about his behavior but did not report it. Tikvah knows of two other women whom the physician has abused sexually, one of them his patient and another a lab technician in the hospital where he worked. He also showed her a list of all the women he had sexual encounters with, dating back to his days as a resident, including a notation of whether they were a nurse or patient and what color hair they had.

In early 1998 Tikvah called her state's Medical Quality Assurance Board to ask if her physician's behavior and that of his colleagues were illegal. She did not give her name, as "I'm paranoid, I don't trust the system." The person she spoke to assured her that the behavior was indeed illegal and begged her to give her name, to break the "collusion of silence." In April she called back and gave her name and was immediately put through to the director, a man. "They shouldn't have had me speak to a man, I should have had the option of having a man or a woman." They said they would be in touch "right away," but it was not until two weeks later that they sent an investigator to talk to her. "For someone in my position, two weeks is a very long time, too long after I finally decided to come forward." The investigator, an older woman, was "wonderful." "I told her the story and gave her the names of the people I knew who knew about it, but who had never reported it." A week later, the investigator sent me a letter saying, "Here's a draft of what you told me," which was inaccurate. Tikvah was upset about that, too. "When you're trying to be heard . . ."

"Once they got my statement, it was a big void. It became an issue of them against the physician." The investigator did keep in touch with her, however, and in fact "broke confidentiality" to tell her what was happening. That also made Tikvah trust the investigator less, even though it made it possible for her to find out what she wanted to know.

"Then I became a person who wasn't even a victim. . . . it was shitty. I became 'the alleged victim.' . . . it was dehumanizing, it could have been any 'body.'" The physician admitted he had sex with her but said that she had wanted it. He never admitted that he had medicated her out of the office, even though there were witnesses to it. "All the stories were told; it finally went before the Board for review to decide if it should go forward for a hearing." The board decided that there was enough evidence to go forward, so it had a hearing, and it was to make a decision in September. September became October while the board obtained more information, and then it referred the case to its legal department. The person who was now in charge of the case told Tikvah, "I can't tell you anything. This physician has rights." Tikvah took this to mean that the physician had more rights than she did.

She finally heard in December, after she had called several times seeking information. By then, when she called, and the legal officer found out who it was, he said, "What do you want? We sent it to the Attorney General's office. You have no right to information, it has nothing to do with you." This resulted in a shouting match between the two: "I went Kamikaze," said Tikvah. She told the officer that if she had a lawyer, he wouldn't be treated this way, to which the officer replied, "At least the attorney wouldn't be histrionic." He corrected her use of the word "charges," substituting the word "allegations." "*You* don't get to decide if they are charges or not." In the end Tikvah was unable to obtain information from him and called the supervisor, who oversaw the program. She was very empathic. "He just doesn't get it, he's a man." For Tikvah this made the situation even worse, as if, she said, "anyone who has a phallus cannot be trusted."

The board finally charged the physician with sexual abuse and "moral turpitude" and served him with the relevant papers. Tikvah is convinced that the board cares more about the latter charge than the former, which also fuels her anger at the board. At this point, she is waiting to hear from the board about his response to the charges; he had 20 days to respond and could ask for an extra 60 days. "The board promised to tell me [what happened]; they didn't. If he loses his license, I'd be shocked." The board is supposed to place such charges on its Web site even before a decision, to inform the public; it has not done so. Tikvah's calls to find out why have gone unanswered.

Tikvah is also angry at the legal profession; she called 40 attorneys trying to find one who would take the case. They told her that the statute of limitations had expired, for which she blamed them for delaying in their offers to represent her. She also wants them to challenge the statute of limitations, as the lawyer she finally found is planning to do. At the moment, her lawyer and the lawyers for the physician and the insurance company are in the typical back-and-forth, which Tikvah also interprets as meaning that they are all unreliable. "I'm paranoid; I don't trust the system," she says again. She is not happy with the lawyer who is currently representing her. "My once supportive attorney is no longer as supportive now that he has learned that the doctor's insurance company can probably not be held accountable for paying what they consider 'intentional' abuse. He was very blunt that he was working on a case 'worth several million' and would deal with my case as he 'had time.' This same attorney is not interested in suing the local hospital even though I was raped there—and he constantly tells me that his firm is not supportive of suing a Catholic hospital. He also spoke of how 'it is a small town and there is a lot of political pressure here' and he suggested that I get a grip and 'understand that no other lawyer would take your case but we are doing you a favor.'"

Why These Problems Exist

Tikvah's case is an excellent example of the problems inherent in such cases. A person who complains needs the kind of support the board is not in a position to provide. Its interests are different, and it does not represent the victim. Tikvah is suffering from the same alienation as many rape victims who do not understand their relatively minor role in the case against the defendant. Just as is the case here, the victim is not the central figure, but merely a witness. Like many rape victims, she is very hurt by what looks to her like the minimizing of her suffering by those involved in processing the complaint against the physician. She is outraged to hear that the physician has rights. From her point of view, after all he has done to her and considering what a danger she perceives him to be, he does not deserve any legal protection. Given her psychological state, events and statements that might otherwise seem neutral are full of negative meaning to her. Her dealings with the board reflect this mistrust and anger, which perhaps is why it no longer answers her calls; it may well perceive her as crazy, hysterical, and therefore impossible to deal with. The pattern is repeated with her lawyer, which adds to her feeling of being marginalized and put down, which in turn adds to her "paranoia."

Most of the other victims I have interviewed have sounded much calmer in their descriptions of their encounters with regulatory agencies, even those who did not have a good experience. It may be that they had already worked through their anger and could in retrospect describe the events in what we consider dispassionate, neutral terms. Success in dealing with regulatory agencies is likely to be connected to the extent that a woman who complains can come across as calm and dispassionate. Otherwise, she risks receiving the classic female label of the hysterical woman whose story is suspect. Once she is so labeled, as Tikvah evidently was, a regulatory agency will be less willing to provide her with the information and support that she so clearly needs. This, in turn, contributes to the belief on the part of victims that the complaint process is revictimizing, and this, in turn, discourages others from complaining.

The Model Case

In contrast to most of the other cases described to me, P. E.'s case is a textbook example of the good victim and the good board. Her abuser was involved in boundary violations for a period of eight years and sexual behavior for six months. While she was still seeing him, she started seeing another therapist, who believed her immediately when she told him of the sexual misconduct. Together they worked to arrange a face-to-face encounter with the abusing therapist, which she describes as "very affirming." Because she "didn't hear things from him that I wanted to hear," P. E. decided to file with the State Board of Psychology, even though he basically admitted the abuse during that encounter. She prepared a very detailed and "dispassionate" document in support of her complaint. She mailed the complaint and supporting document on a Friday, and by the following Tuesday she had been contacted by the board's investigator, who said that this case was being given priority because of its egregious nature. Within ten days, he got permission from the board to do a full investigation and had a detailed interview with P. E. a few days later. The investigator was very skilled at interviewing her and was "very polite, very kind." The case appeared so clear that the board, in fact, mailed the document in which they suspended the abuser's license the day before the interview. This was an emergency suspension, to be followed by revocation, unless the therapist appeals. Unlike most boards, this particular board is required to revoke the license of someone who has been proved to have engaged in sexual misconduct.

This case is very unusual both in the speed and in the seriousness with which the complaint was addressed. P. E. thinks it had a lot to do with her credibility. As a professional writer, she was able to write the document in support of her complaint with great care. She has also had the help of an excellent subsequent therapist, "who did everything right. He has been an excellent advocate." Her current therapist was also able to support P. E.'s claim, as he was present at the face-to-face encounter and heard the abuser say that he agreed with P. E.'s claim. All the elements described here combine to make this a good case: a calm, dispassionate victim, a supportive and knowledgeable subsequent therapist, and a board that listens to victims and takes serious action fast.

Understanding the Process

Another problem is that many victims do not understand other aspects of the process. As required by law, boards are concerned for the due process rights of the professional, who is at risk of losing his livelihood. Courts have recognized that professional licenses are property rights and that, therefore, boards have a constitutional obligation not to take them away without due process (Bisbing et al., 1995: 865–70). For this reason the professional has a variety of rights: to notice, to a fair and impartial hearing, to counsel to represent him, to confrontation and cross-examination, to protection against self-incrimination, and to a record of the proceedings. This is why the victim has to tell her story over and over again to those investigating the case as well as those hearing it. It is also why her story is very likely to be questioned by the lawyer for the professional, behavior that looks to her as if, once again, she is not being believed. It is also why in K's case, described earlier, she had to leave at the end of her testimony, but "he got to stay." It is also why the proceedings are not made public until after formal charges have been filed. The need for careful investigation, combined with the backlogs caused by the perennial lack of funding for the boards, contributes to the delays, which look to the victim like negligence and bias in favor of the professional. Because the charges have not yet been legally proved, unless the professional can be persuaded to surrender his license voluntarily, he can continue to practice for the two or three years these cases often take; just as in a criminal case, he is innocent until proven guilty. It is also why it is difficult, though not impossible, to charge a professional unless there is specific wording prohibiting the behavior.

In Vicki's case, the complaint was about posttermination sex, but the board could not act because the code of conduct did not refer to "former clients." "As luck would have it, the perpetrator and his lawyer found out that the WV [West Virginia] state code did not refer to the new updated code of ethics for social workers which is specific on exactly what a social worker can and cannot do. . . . I had been out of treatment a whole month when sexual intercourse began! . . . and the old code left ethical standards with former clients up to the individual counselor. Well, this jewel got off with a warning. He has lived with clients, dated other clients, and recently married a client!" (Campbell, 1999). The board had received many verbal complaints about this professional, though Vicki's had been the first written complaint. It is possible that the board could have taken more serious action than giving a warning by applying general ethical requirements for the profession, though in doing so, it ran a significant risk of having its decision appealed. It therefore erred on the side of caution, behavior that did not vindicate Vicki in her complaint. Her dissatisfaction was tempered somewhat by the fact that the board "did manage to get the legislative code changed too late to help with my case," but Vicki was told there were a couple of other complaints that were to be tried under the new rule.

From the Other Side: The Professional's Perspective

It is ironic that professionals and victims complain about many of the same things in the way cases are handled by the various boards (Schoener, 1 March 1999). The Committee on Physician Sexual Misconduct in British Columbia reports that patients and physicians alike complain of long delays in which they have no idea what is happening (*Crossing the Boundaries*, 1992: 72). The delay has different, but potentially damaging, effects on both professionals and victims. For a victim, there is no closure while the case drags on. For a professional to have his reputation in question and his life on hold for several years can be psychologically and financially devastating. Both victims and professionals complain that the boards often do not have the facts accurately presented. They both complain about the expense; many victims cannot afford to hire a lawyer to represent them at the hearing, though this can be very supportive and helpful. Professionals must hire a lawyer, which can drain their entire life savings, especially as many of them do not have malpractice insurance for licensing board complaints.

Some professionals argue that they are hounded by licensing authorities, denied due process, and considered guilty of the charge until they can prove their innocence. In an effort to protect themselves and provide information to professionals as well as to lobby for changes in the law and board procedure, they have formed an organization called Professional Advocacy Network (PAN). It was founded several years ago by a psychologist, Dr. Lynn Steinberg in California, because she was appalled by the way her case was conducted by the Board of Psychology (Steinberg, 1997).

PAN claims that it has been in touch with people who have been badly treated by licensing boards all over the country and has many members lobbying for legislative changes. Like all these organizations, it is chronically short of money and is therefore unable to do much apart from give advice. It had one conference in April 1996 and has lobbied for changes in the law in California, so far unsuccessfully (Steinberg, 1999). When asked about membership numbers, Dr. Steinberg defined members as those with whom they had been in touch, which numbered then at over 6,000 (Steinberg, 1997). The number of actual dues-paying membership is much lower, in part, according to Steinberg, because the professionals are "bankrupted" by the licensing procedures so that they cannot afford the dues. Most of their members are psychologists, with a liberal sprinkling of lawyers, "many of whom are mercenary, but some are also very concerned" about the plight of professionals (Steinberg, 1997).

According to Steinberg, the number of members is directly related to how "bad" the state boards are, which she defines as those states that have the highest number of complaints brought. The state with the highest rate is Oregon, followed by New York, California, Texas, and Arizona (Steinberg, 1997). Certain kinds of professionals appear to be the most vulnerable; in psychology, it is those who practice in the humanist tradition and who do not hold to the tight boundary rules of other members of the profession. Professionals who use other, nontraditional methods are also vulnerable. Steinberg said that she had never heard of a Freudian being disciplined. In medicine, those who practice alternative medicine are likely to be brought before the board. It appears also that people defined as "troublemakers" for the boards are also likely targets. Gary Schoener, the leader in the field of professional sexual misconduct, has had several run-ins with his state board, based on its (inaccurate) perception that he claims he has a Ph.D. when, in fact, he does not (Schoener, 1 March 1999). Andrew Kane, another psychologist who has done extensive research in the field of professional sexual misconduct, has been involved in charges by the Wisconsin Board of Psychologists for several years. The board hired a consultant, whose recommendation it did not like, so it hired another expert, at great expense to both Kane and the taxpayers (Schoener, 1 March 1999).

PAN has a number of claims about what is wrong with the current procedures. It argues that boards are overzealous and conduct secret investigations, often by ex-cops who know nothing about the profession, behind the back of the professional being investigated. They believe that due process is also denied in the power of those states where the board can overrule the determination of administrative hearings, even on an appellate level. The professional suffers terrible professional damage, even if he or she is found not guilty of the charges. In part, this is because if a board decides this is an emergency, it can suspend the license immediately, which gives the professional no time to make arrangements for patients, either for the duration of the hearing process or for the duration of the suspension. Patients are thus left without adequate care, which, ironically, is itself a violation of professional ethics. It is also because—PAN members believe—some boards have overreacted to the recent concern about sexual misconduct to the point that they believe that the professional is guilty until proven innocent. In California, if the charges are proven, the board is required to suspend the professional's license. The costs of defending oneself against the charges are so great, they argue, that many professionals are forced to negotiate a plea because they cannot afford to prove their innocence. They also argue that, in fact, this is not "peer" regulation at all but a small clique of professionals who stand in judgment over all the various branches of the professions about whom they are not experts—nor are the "experts" who testify regularly in the hearing process.

One Professional's Story

Dr. Donald Crowe has been involved in the complaint process with the California Board of Psychology since an ex-patient filed a complaint against him in August 1991 (Crowe, 1998). The complainant was a woman with whom he had a posttermination sexual relationship in 1990. He says that the complaint was filed after he refused to marry the woman. The board filed a formal accusation late in 1994, and a hearing was held in March 1995. After two weeks of trial, the administrative law judge found him innocent of sexual misconduct and recommended a probationary period and an oral reexamination for boundary violations, such as finishing lunch in front of the patient prior to a session. The board decided not to adopt the judge's findings and revoked his license on 15 February 1996. It gave him two days to terminate over 50 patients. The Superior Court of Alameda County granted a stay of revocation and then ordered the board to reconsider its decision in light of many mitigating circumstances. The board revoked his license again on 25 February 1997. The Superior Court overturned the board again, ordering it to stop charging him with sexual misconduct. The board met with Crowe on 22 August 1997 for "oral argument" and then revoked his license, this time for "gross negligence." At this point Crowe's legal fees were over $400,000. The Superior Court overturned the board yet again, this time charging it with six instances of "manifestly gross abuse of discretion" and ordered a penalty less than revocation. Finally, on 16 January 1998 the board and Crowe arrived at a stipulated agreement amounting to limited conditions of probation.

While Crowe's battle with the California Board of Psychology is now finally over, the American Psychological Association is now taking up its investigation to determine whether he is fit to be a member of the professional association (Crowe, 1999). We examine this remedy in the next section.

This case is the most extreme one of which I have heard, but it does illustrate several more widespread problems with the system. The case has dragged on for a number of years, causing psychological trauma and financial disaster. Dr. Crowe's professional life has suffered what may be irretrievable damage. The expenses to the taxpayers of pursuing this case would be greater than in the usual case, but nevertheless, the costs are always high. The case also illustrates the possibility of abuse of discretion by an administrative agency. It may be that the Board of Psychology believes that it is responding to the demand for greater accountability, but in this case it is at the expense of the life of one practitioner. As one lawyer who practices in this field said about sexual misconduct, "[T]he Board seeks revocation, will go to the mat for revocation" (Radlett-Kollar, 1996).

Follow-Up by Licensing Boards

One of the problems faced by licensing boards is that of monitoring the professionals against whom they have taken action. Boards have broad discretion to determine an appropriate penalty that they believe serves both to punish the professional and to protect the public (Bisbing et al., 1999: 107). As discussed before, boards are usually very unwilling to deprive professionals of their livelihood and therefore attempt to hand down a penalty that falls short of loss of license but works to "rehabilitate" the professional so that he does not reoffend. This goal is reinforced by the fact that it is still possible for a therapist to continue to practice as an unlicensed therapist, even after he has lost his license. In addition, it is possible for a professional to continue to practice in another state, as there is no national system of communication of revocation of licenses from one state to another. Such evidence as there is indicates that both of these events happen (Lehr, 1994: 14; Mooney, 1994; Schoener, 19 April 1995). Thus, licensing boards try to keep some control over those they sanction; they believe that there is a greater chance of rehabilitation if they put together a package in which the professional is required to undergo evaluation, therapy, and education and practice under limited conditions.

This system, although laudable in its intent, does not appear to work so well in practice (Bisbing, 1999: 107–8). It is based on the assumption that sexual misconduct is a curable problem, an assumption not supported by evidence in either this or related areas of offending (Dehlendorf and Wolfe, 1997: 27). Many boards design rehabilitation schemes without much assessment, so it is difficult to determine exactly what they are following up on (Schoener, 1 March 1999). In fact, Schoener argues that real evaluations are extremely rare. Relatively few people in the country are qualified to undertake them, and, of course, they are expensive, so most boards make do with a rather cursory examination. They also often leave the implementation of their order solely to the discretion of an outside "expert" (Bisbing et al., 1999: 108). This is a rather dangerous course, as these offenders are likely to remain in practice, and the risk is, of course, that they will reoffend. I have heard frequently of "punishments" that look laughably inappropriate to the victims and others, as, for example, in the case of a psychologist against whom 48 charges were brought who was ordered to take an ethics course and to retake his oral exam, while still being allowed to practice (Parker, 1999). One therapist was sentenced to 50 hours of continuing medical education, which simply did not exist in the state; the board later admitted that it had sentenced him to something that did not exist (Schoener, 1 March 1999). Another was sentenced to 10 hours, which also did not exist. When told this, the board asked, "Well, can you provide a reading list?," as if reading a few books will stop this behavior (Schoener, 1 March 1999). This is not only a problem in the United States. In New Zealand, which is seen by some as a model in the way it handles complaints of violations of medical ethics, one physician was ordered to take a course in "boundary issues," which did not exist. On appeal to the District Court, the court quashed the order (Urquhart, 1999).

Often, therapy is ordered, but the offender may be allowed to select his own therapist; he is very likely to pick a sympathetic friend rather than someone who is trained to deal with problems of professional sexual misconduct. In addition, because of the absence of evaluation, the conditions of practice ordered by the board may represent myth rather than empirical information about the nature of professional sexual misconduct. One therapist, for example, was allowed to treat only men and older women, on the unverified assumption that he was interested in exploiting only young women. Such a requirement does not take into account the ethical deficiency shown by the professional, which affects his performance generally, not just toward certain groups (Dehlendorf and Wolfe, 1997: 28).

There is another, more basic problem with following up on the cases; it often does not happen. Serious monitoring of conditions of probation demand personnel and time, which many boards simply do not provide. Thus, they have no way of knowing whether the conditions have really been met.

About half the states specify a minimum period, ranging from one to five years after revocation, before restoration is permitted. Even when this happens (and we have seen how rare it is), it appears to be fairly easy to have it reinstated after a short period. Virtually no empirical evidence is available, but interviews with professionals involved in the area indicate that only in the most notorious cases does a professional have his application for reinstatement turned down.

Professional Organizations and the Control of Misconduct

As mentioned earlier, one option available for a victim is to file a complaint with the ethics committee of the appropriate professional organization (Bisbing et al., 1995: 889–94). Empirical data on the actions of professional organizations in the control of their members are even harder to come by than in the case of licensing boards. None of the relevant national organizations (American Psychiatric Association, American Psychological Association, National Association of Social Workers) keep any national statistics of ethics violations. State organizations keep either no information at all or only statistics for all types of misconduct without breaking them down by type of behavior.

Complaining to the local professional organization is listed on the "Wheel of Options" mentioned at the beginning of this chapter. It is also presented as one option in the brochures put out by various organizations, both public and private, on the subject of professional sexual misconduct, though the brochure published in 1999 by the Maryland Department of Health and Mental Hygiene does not include a complaint to a professional association in its list of steps a victim can take (*Broken Boundaries*, 1999: 7). In fact, provision of such a brochure to someone who alleges professional sexual misconduct is required by California law (Cal. Bus. & Prof. Code s.723 [a] [West 1990]). What most victims are not told, however, is that it is really an empty remedy, although some experts now advise complainants not to bother with ethics committees (Schoener, 6 November 1995; Wohlberg, 1998). The rate of success is minuscule, the process is elongated, and the pressures mitigating against any significant penalty are so great that it is hardly worth the time and emotional investment a victim must put in. As one victim put it, "I did want to contact the American Psychiatric Association. . . . however I had been through so much. . . . I didn't have the emotional energy to follow through with a complaint. . . . Rather than contacting the APA, which has very little power, I would rather use my energy through advocacy." Professionals who work with victims maintain that they hear more complaints about ethics committees' handling of complaints than any other process (Wohlberg, 1998). One victim described the process to me as "the dumbest waste of time." This view is supported by Luepker's (1999) research, in which her respondents were less likely to be satisfied with the outcome of their complaint to a professional organization than to a regulatory board.

Even if a complaint is successful, the only remedies available to the association are reprimand, suspension, and termination from membership (Bisbing et al., 1995: 891–92). While being licensed is required in many professions, membership in the relevant professional organization is not, which seriously limits the power of the organization to sanction its members. Some associations publish the names of the offending member in their association newsletter, which may give the actions a bit more force ("Sexual Exploitation," 1996: 90).

I was told several times that a member who feels under threat of an ethics complaint hearing need only resign, and the organization no longer has any authority to pursue the matter. The psychiatrist whose case was the subject of the *Firing Line* program resigned from the Colorado Psychiatric Association, alleging that he could not afford the dues ("My

Doctor, My Lover," 1993). When the association offered to waive them, he offered another reason for resigning. There was no ethics hearing in that case, and he is still practicing psychiatry, even though he lost the civil lawsuit (Roberts, 26 October 1995). Even if the member does not resign, the strongest action available is termination from membership, which is hardly a significant punishment, although that may be less true now as more insurance companies are asking insurance applicants whether they are members of their professional associations. For some professionals, not being a member means not being eligible for some malpractice insurance policies.

What does seem to be happening is that some professional ethics committees no longer handle serious cases or even any cases, but refer complainants to the licensing authorities (Schoener, 6 November 1995). About half of state psychology associations ethics committees no longer hear complaints, though such committees are being set up in other disciplines (Clarke and Barnett, 1998). In the survey of all state psychological associations, an additional 12 of the associations were planning changes, most of which were in the direction of eliminating or reducing their investigative role (Clarke and Barnett, 1998: 5). It is ironic that this is happening at a time when outside forces are actually increasing their power over members. Recently, insurance companies have been asking professionals who want malpractice insurance whether they have been the subject of an ethics committee complaint. If a prospective insured has had a complaint, he or she might not be able to get insurance, an outcome that is much more likely if the prospective insured has had an adverse outcome (Schoener, 6 November 1995). Complaints and negative hearing outcomes may also have to be reported to health maintenance organizations, which might result in loss of income or not being permitted to practice for that organization (Wohlberg, 1998).

The most important issue here is not how much power the professional association has but the way in which it is willing to exercise it. While the organizations may say that they are consumer-oriented, evidence would belie this view, and it is clear that they are less consumer-oriented than licensing boards. Their role is more of a guild to protect the interests of their members, and thus they are structurally unsuitable for the task of self-policing. As one expert put it: "It is like asking the fox to guard the henhouse" (Schoener, 6 November 1995). There are, however, legitimate reasons ethics committees are no longer hearing complaints. They see a conflict between providing advice and guidance to their members about complaints and hearing the complaints themselves. They also see their efforts as a duplication of the process conducted by licensing boards, which are perceived to be both better equipped for the task and more likely to be seen as neutral and concerned with protecting the public (Wohlberg, 1998). Many groups have changed their focus to one in which they advise their members who have had licensing complaints filed against them and refer complaints they receive to the appropriate licensing board ("Sexual Exploitation," 1996: 90). The reason most associations gave for discontinuing their investigative role was, however, the fear of liability, a specter we have seen elsewhere in this area and in others (e.g., Bohmer and Parrot, 1993; Clarke and Barnett, 1998: 5). That this fear is, in fact, unrealistic is borne out by evidence that there have been only seven threatened lawsuits against state psychological associations ever (Clarke and Barnett, n.d.: 8).

These changes are reflected in the number of victims who are willing to file an ethics committee complaint. Virtually none of the victims I interviewed in the last several years had filed such a complaint; the typical response was a civil suit and a licensing board complaint.

COOPERATION AMONG THE VARIOUS REGULATORY AGENCIES

One of the central tenets of professional self-regulation is that control of misconduct is the responsibility of the profession itself. The professional associations and licensing authorities rely, in part, on the profession to report incidents of misconduct, especially since, it is argued, it is in the best position to determine whether particular behavior is likely to be misconduct. It is striking, therefore, how little connection there appears to be among the various organizations responsible for the control of professional behavior. We saw in the previous chapter that few of the criminal cases were the result of reports from other professionals or agencies; the majority of complaints on which criminal cases were based came from victims. The lack of contact works the other way, also. In Kane's (1995) study of the criminalization of therapist–patient sex, he found that only three district attorney respondents reported giving any information to the licensing boards for physicians or psychologists (319).

In an effort to deal with the paucity of reports, six states have passed mandatory reporting laws under which a therapist who has reason to believe that a colleague has sexually exploited a patient is required to report it (Bisbing et al., 1998: 12). There is not much information about the extent to which this increases the rate of reporting in the United States. Preliminary figures in Ontario, which also recently instituted a mandatory reporting law for physicians, indicated that it does have an effect on the reporting rate. Before the mandatory provision came into effect, the rate of reporting by members of the profession was 6 per month; the rate jumped to 22 per month since the mandatory reporting law came into effect (Dempsey, 1994). Dempsey explains the position of the reporting physician as follows: "Those physicians who report generally find the task of doing so disagreeable, but are for the most part relieved that mandatory reporting means they do not have to make a judgment about reporting a colleague for alleged sexual abuse. The decision of whether or not to pursue the matter becomes the responsibility of the College" (23). In fact, the responsibility has always been with the licensing board, in this case the College of Physicians and Surgeons. Apparently, doctors are now more willing to let it take the responsibility without feeling guilt at turning in a colleague.

The different methods of controlling professional sexual misconduct described have not been set up to be interconnected. But it is hard not to see them as connected in that they are all efforts to address the same problem. Cooperation among the different mechanisms would, therefore, have a salutary effect both on the handling of complaints and on the incidence of the misconduct. For example, a criminal conviction provides a strong foundation for action by the professional licensing boards. In some contexts, it is sufficient for some licensing action, and in others, it provides excellent evidence of misconduct. That some boards do not seem too enthusiastic to use the criminal conviction is illustrated by the case of a doctor who was found guilty of raping an anesthetized woman he was treating for back pain. The New York state officials decided to wait until he was sentenced, on the ground that his guilt was not official until then! In New Jersey, where the doctor also practiced, his license was suspended much earlier ("Our Sleeping Doctor Watchers," 1995).

This cooperation would also be effective between professional organizations and licensing authorities. Given what we have seen about the limitations of the ethics board hearings by professional associations, it makes sense for those organizations to be in close cooperation with those who do have power over the professionals. It appears that many ethics boards of professional organizations no longer hear complaints themselves but instead refer complainants to the licensing authorities (Schoener, 6 November 1995). In one study of state psychological associations, 17 percent of the responding states actually were required by statute to pass complaints to the relevant licensing board (Clarke and Barnett, 1998: 12). Interestingly, 23 percent of the respondents, virtually all of whom were either the executive director or ethics chair, were unsure of their statutory obligations. For example, in California, if the association disciplines a psychologist, it is obliged to notify the board of examiners, while in South Dakota, all complaints go to the board. The Maryland Psychiatric Society refers all complaints to the Maryland Board of Physician Quality Assurance, which "investigates cases, assigns them for peer review . . . and develops consent orders involving sanctions. Our Ethics Committee then works with the statement of facts from the consent agreement, and with any additional consideration provided by the psychiatrist, to decide on a membership sanction" (Bunes, 1994). Bunes, the executive director of the Maryland Psychological Association, points out that since these procedures (which, in fact, are mandated by the Maryland Medical Practice Act) have been adopted, every case has resulted in a serious membership sanction. Some states refer complaints routinely even in the absence of a statutory obligation, for example, Virginia (Clarke and Barnett, 1998: 12).

Licensing boards do seem to be using the results of civil suits as a basis for their actions. I have interviewed a number of victims who have told me that the licensing board put the case on hold until after the civil suit is settled or tried. Either result buttresses the board's claim of misconduct and diminishes the chance of a long and costly appeal of its decision.

In addition to providing information to assist other authorities in the control of professional sexual misconduct, cooperation would have the benefit of increasing the publicity surrounding the problem. While professionals deny that they want to hide cases of sexual misconduct, the way the system is set up has this effect. Associations and licensing boards vary in how readily available they make information about their actions. A consumer could probably find out if a professional had been sanctioned by his association or his licensing board if she knew how to investigate; however, it is not easy and is often not published anywhere. If one of the goals of these various different methods of controlling professional sexual misconduct is deterring other professionals from engaging in such conduct, then this lack of information hardly helps in securing that goal. Thus, even if there is no conscious effort to deny information to the public about the conduct of professionals in this area, the effect of the system is to do just that. The deterrent value of such publicity on would-be sexual exploiters is lost as long as they do not know of the punishments of others.

THE ROLE OF CONSUMERS

One of the problems with professional self-regulation is that it does not take into account the role of the consumers of professional services. As we have become a more consumer-oriented society, this lack has become more apparent. Yet the agencies that control professional behavior have been very slow to respond to consumer demands for greater input into the regulatory process. For example, most medical boards have at least one lay member, but that is not usually sufficient to "counteract the self-protective impulses of the medical profession" (Dehlendorf and Wolfe, 1997: 29). Many commentators have recommended a greater consumer role in the disciplining of professionals. Dehlendorf and Wolfe, in their report, suggest that much more public representation is needed. "More well-trained consumer representatives, selected based on a history of advocacy for patients, must be integrated into all medical boards, for only then will physicians be held to the standards of conduct and competence expected by patients and society, rather than by the overly lenient perspectives of many of their colleagues" (29).

Other countries have taken a different approach. In New Zealand and some states in Australia, for example, there is a separate government agency to represent consumers in cases of complaints against professionals. In 1996 New Zealand appointed a health and disability commissioner to deal with all health-related consumer complaints. While those who work in the system are not yet satisfied with its current functioning, it does have the advantage of providing monitoring of the profession by outsiders, rather than by the profession itself (Urquhart, 1999).

Whatever changes take place, they are more likely to come from consumers rather than the profession itself. The Maryland Task Force Report remarked on this: "[T]he biggest incentive for change has come from consumer advocates" ("Sexual Exploitation," 1996).

CONCLUSION

We have seen in this chapter how difficult it is to determine what proportion of cases of misconduct results in any action by criminal or regulatory authorities. It is abundantly clear that in only a minuscule proportion is any official action taken. On paper, someone who alleges professional sexual misconduct has an unusually large range of options available, especially when compared with those abused in other ways, like rape and domestic violence. In reality, however, these options are unlikely to result in an outcome satisfactory to the victim, nor can they do much to reduce the incidence of professional sexual misconduct.

The reasons for the low rate of action are many and varied. Both victims and professionals are reluctant to complain, and professional organizations and licensing boards are underfunded and often not trained to carry out the investigation required. Increasingly, the whole process has become more legalistic, which only makes it more cumbersome and adds to the costs and the delays involved.

The argument that only professionals can evaluate the behavior of their colleagues is much less valid in cases of sexual misconduct where fact-finding and credibility are the central issues rather than appropriate medical practice. These issues might be better handled within the court system, which has the relevant expertise. It could be argued that even if it were a matter of professional practice, the courts are better equipped, with the help of experts, to make such judgments. Ironically, as so many of these cases end up in court anyway, the regulatory system may be, to some extent, duplicating the work of the court.

Professionals have a strong interest in continuing to control the system themselves. It might also be argued that they have an interest in keeping the details of the system as secret as possible, to minimize the negative publicity about such professional misconduct. The way the system is set up, however, and the way records are kept make it exceedingly difficult to get a clear picture of exactly what is going on. There is tremendous variation among the states both in the proportion of cases handled and in the efficiency of the record keeping.

The shift from professional control to the criminal control described in the last chapter is best seen as a change in orientation and the goals of the system rather than a way of increasing the proportion of professionals whose behavior results in some negative state action. As we have seen, very few prosecutions take place in those states that have criminal statutes. But a criminal response does represent a move away from professional control to community control, as well as a shift to an emphasis on punishment as a means of protecting the public. As one respondent from the Board of Medical Practice put it: "Our mission . . . is the protection of the public. It is not punishment of miscreants, vengeance or any such actions" (Martz, 1995). While Dr. Martz believes that his agency's methods of psychiatric treatment, suspension of license, and supervised practice have been effective, others argue that the criminal law can provide more effective control (Schoener, 6 November 1995). For example, only a judge can make an offender refrain from practicing without a license in his state or in another state by making it a condition of probation. Increased consumer input might change the way the agencies operate and increase the protection of the public rather than the profession. Thus, who controls the system affects how the control is exercised and whose interests are represented. The current system does not appear to be very effective in controlling the problem of professional sexual misconduct.

—9—

PROFESSIONAL SEXUAL MISCONDUCT AS A SOCIAL MOVEMENT

INTRODUCTION

In this chapter, I discuss professional sexual exploitation as a social movement in an effort to explain why it has not been much of a success, especially when compared to other social movements. In addition to comparing professional sexual exploitation with other social movements, I use the relevant scholarship on social movements as a source of explanation for what we have seen in previous chapters.

THE DEFINITION OF SUCCESS

Whether a movement is a success depends on how it is defined. If the movement is defined in readily identifiable terms, it is much easier to say whether it has been a success or not. For example, from Nelson's (1984) analysis, the passage of child abuse legislation throughout the country can be judged a tremendous success as long as it is defined in terms of legislative change. The success of this movement was in the nationwide change in the child abuse laws, which drew attention to the subject and began the system of requiring the reporting of incidents of suspected child abuse by various professionals. Nelson did not address the effect this public attention and legal activity had on the incidence of child abuse. A further example of success, defined in terms of legislative change, is in Jacob's (1988) study of divorce law reform. He documents how every state rewrote its divorce law in a relatively short period in the 1970s and early 1980s. So dramatic does he consider this change that he calls his book *Silent Revolution*. Divorce itself, however, is no less of a problem now. In fact, some argue that the divorce law reform movement has caused the current problems with divorce.[1] What was "revolutionary," according to Jacob, was the change in the way divorce was perceived by the law, from a system based on marital fault to one based on marital breakdown.

Another interesting case of definition-driven success is the rape reform movement. When it is defined as a movement to reform the rape laws to have a major beneficial impact in the legal conduct of a rape trial, it has been shown to be a failure (Berger et al., 1988; Loh, 1981). If, on the other hand, it is defined more broadly, it could be defined as a success: it has heightened public awareness, changed attitudes somewhat, increased the willingness of women to report, and made their treatment by the criminal justice system a little more sensitive (Spohn and Horney, 1992; Bourque, 1989). Similarly, the movement for tort reform has been very successful in changing the behavior of juries, which have accepted the arguments made by interest group ad campaigns and widespread dissemination of the belief that plaintiffs sue to get rich and do not deserve much compensation for their injuries (Daniels et al., 1999). This success has been much more significant in lowering jury awards than any actual tort reform legislation that the media campaign was designed to achieve.

The most extreme divergence in definitions of success might be in Johnston's (1980) piece on the success of transcendental meditation (TM) as a social movement. Johnston specifically describes the movement as a success, as measured evidently by number of adherents; however, he describes the goals of the movement as world peace and universal happiness. It would be hard to find a movement with goals less likely to be realized than these!

As in all social movements, those concerned about professional sexual misconduct do not all share the same goals. Some of them are interested in catching individual perpetrators, some want the church to acknowledge its part in the problem, some are looking to various kinds of legislation as a solution, some want education of professionals and better regulatory control, and some want to stop the problem. The "success" of the professional sexual misconduct movement varies depending on which of these goals one uses in the definition. While the problem has by no means been stopped, and there is little evidence that it has even been reduced significantly, there have been a number of legislative successes, increased regulatory attention, and increased professional awareness.

Success also depends on who is doing the defining. While some activists in the movement acknowledge that the time for maximum public interest has passed despite the continued existence of the problem, those on the "other side" of the movement, for example, the clergy, are behaving as if the problem, though it did once exist, has been dealt with and is therefore no longer of any concern (SNAP Conference, 1996).

Another factor in the definition of success is the question of timing. While arguments that something failed because "the time was not right" have a way of becoming circular, one can say that efforts to regulate professional sexual misconduct have come up against the roadblock of the antiregulation mood of the times (Hux, 1995). This, of course, may be a justification by those who do not want legal and regulatory control of this particular behavior. After all, the efforts to criminalize professional sexual misconduct are the major current activism effort in this area, and no one could argue that reluctance to add regulations has limited current changes in other areas of the criminal law when legislatures respond with alacrity to publicity about a huge variety of social problems by passing laws. Another element of the timing issue is that success itself is time-based. Today's failure may be tomorrow's success, a fact that makes the determination of whether something is a success or not rather difficult. It can also work the other way: the more successful the movement is in precipitating a particular social change, the less successful it is likely to be as a permanent organization (Eyerman and Jamison, 1991). This connects back to the framing of the problem itself. Some movements—or, at least, organizations—have ensured their durability by reframing the issue once the original problem has been solved. The March of Dimes is an example of this; having solved the problem for which it was formed (polio), it then engaged in domain expansion and reframed itself as an organization that deals with a variety of childhood diseases. Other movements may be framed in ways that make them unlikely ever to succeed; the rape reform movement will never stamp out rape, for example, nor will the battered woman's movement eliminate domestic violence.

FRAMING PROBLEMS

For a movement to be successful, it is necessary, among other things, for it to obtain support for its views and to prod those people into action who already agree with those views (Klandermans, 1984). Snow and Benford (1988) expand on this to describe core framing tasks that need to be fulfilled for a movement to mobilize successfully. Their first framing task involves identifying a problem and attributing blame or causality. This diagnostic framing appears to be relatively easy in the examples used by Snow and Benford. In the case of professional sexual misconduct, even the diagnosis and its cause are the subject of some disagreement. Whether "the problem" involves only adults, whether it involves only women, whether it involves only the therapeutic professions or includes others such as the clergy, lawyers, or academics are all disputed in the framing of professional sexual exploitation. Explanations of blame or causality vary, too. Is it the problem of those victims who get themselves into the situation in the first place? Is this a problem of individual offenders whose behavior itself can be the subject of therapy and "cure"? Is it the problem of the professions themselves, which are not controlling the behavior of their members sufficiently? Or is it the problem of a patriarchal power structure that plays itself out in the professional relationship? This difficulty in finding a cohesive framework has been documented in several chapters of this book.

It is not only at Snow and Benford's first stage of framing that professional sexual exploitation has not succeeded. The second stage, prognostic framing, is also subject to disagreement among framers. They do not agree as to the best "strategies, tactics and targets" (Snow and Benford, 1988: 201). As we have seen, the movement is fragmented among activists who pursue a variety of different strategies. Some stress the need to find and prosecute criminally those offenders so they cannot offend again; others see education as the most beneficial strategy; others are involved in pressing for legal or institutional change. Each of these strategies has a different goal and different targets, and lack of agreement about goals and targets results in a fragmentation of the movement.

Snow and Benford's third core framing task is motivational framing, in which a rationale for action is presented. We have seen that the professional sexual misconduct movement does attempt to inspire people to act to "solve the problem" at meetings and conferences as well as through informal channels. The ability to gather activists and to inspire them to become activists is, however, impeded by the particular nature of the problem itself.

McCarthy (1994), in his case study of drunk driving, shows how important the "proper" interpretation of events is to the mobilizing groups. "But events like auto fatalities must be properly interpreted to be motivating, and proper interpretations must resonate with existing communities of discourse before they can effectively orient collective action" (134). It appears that this has not yet happened in the case of professional sexual misconduct. This may be because of the diverse frames and also because of the ambivalence about the nature and extent of the problem. Many people do not believe that professional sexual misconduct between adults should be framed as a social problem at all, but rather as consensual sexual activity. It is only that part of the problem of child sexual abuse by the clergy about which the public is unambivalent. Connected to this ambivalence is the fact that this is an issue that appears to make people uncomfortable. So, far from being encouraged to engage in collective action, those connected to it, especially many professionals themselves, would rather behave as if the problem does not exist. Other forms of exploitation against women, like rape and domestic violence, have had more success in overcoming this discomfort, perhaps, in part, because they are not issues directed against the very professionals who would otherwise be expected to be central players in fighting it.

For professional sexual misconduct to succeed as an effectively framed social problem, it requires "fairly self-contained but substantial changes in the way a particular domain of social life is framed, such that a domain previously taken for granted is reframed as problematic, and in need of repair" (Snow et al., 1986). As we saw in Chapter 2, those involved in reframing the problem are clearly trying to do just this but do not yet appear to have succeeded with large parts of the domain.

It is not that insufficient sufferers of this problem affect its lack of centrality and consequent "success." As we saw earlier, all the data indicate that the incidence of this problem is widespread in the helping professions. While it is difficult to make statistical comparisons, other social problems do not significantly affect more people and yet have more public salience (see, e.g., the case study of drunk driving: McCarthy, 1994).

CONFLICTS IN THE MOVEMENT: THE INDIVIDUAL VERSUS SOCIAL ACTIVISM

What distinguishes this movement from many others is that it is a combination of individual recovery (healing) and activism for social and legal change. To a large extent, these two goals are in conflict. As we have seen, many of those in the movement are not, in fact, working for social change but for personal change. Many of the issues in this movement that mitigate in favor of healing work against mobilization for collective action. This dichotomy of interests stands in the way of the development of a collective identity (Klandermans, 1992).

A further source of conflict is that in making the claim that this is a major problem that must be taken seriously, victims must show how badly they have suffered and continue to suffer. Psychological trauma is not self-evident in the way bruises from domestic violence are. In addition, such extensive personal suffering as a result of a trauma does not provide the impetus for action that collective movements need to succeed. Only when individual victims move beyond personal suffering can they develop the anger that so often leads people to collective action. But moving beyond suffering risks the implication that the trauma was not so bad after all. Also, many of those who do "recover" from the trauma do so by putting the whole business behind them; this also mitigates against collective action.

For many individuals who are the potential members of the movement, the development of a new identity, that of "survivor," is seen as a central element in the recovery process, as is also the case for victims of other crimes, like rape and domestic violence. That identity is, however, different from, and may conflict with, the identity of "activist" and is not likely to contribute to the success of the movement to change the acceptance and regulation of professional sexual misconduct. In the same way, the nature of the problem itself stands in the way of the development of a social identity that parallels the individual identity. In various ways, the victims of professional sexual misconduct are not what Christie (1986) would call "ideal victims." For many, victims of professional sexual misconduct are actually consenting adults who "had an affair" with the professional that turned sour. Like public attitudes about domestic violence, many believe that the relationship must have been consensual; otherwise, the victim would have walked away from it. Thus, a major issue is the difficulty inherent in defining the events as a problem in the first place (on an individual level) and on a social level (whether it should be a feminist issue or a medical/professional one). The rape reform movement and the domestic violence movement have also struggled with a similar framing problem. One of the marks of the success of those two movements has been their ability to move the frame away from one of individual consensual behavior ("she must have wanted it") to one of unjustified violence against women on a group level.

In addition to this conflict, there are conflicts inherent in the efforts to expand the framing of the problem to include a variety of victims. Differences among the kinds of victims mitigate against the development of an umbrella social identity. Klein (1987) points out that in the case of feminism, the new identity of "women as workers" instead of "women as mothers" does not itself lead to political activism, but it does create new standards for social comparison. Comparing women workers to other workers and then deciding that they were treated unjustly led to political activism. To engage in collective action, people must believe that such action can eliminate their grievances and also that their contribution will affect that success (Klandermans, 1992). For many victims of professional sexual misconduct, either the effort to engage in collective action is more than they can cope with psychologically, or they do not hold out sufficient hope that they can change a system in which so much power is held by the source of the grievance, the professions. Thus, the movement cannot mobilize sufficient resources to engage in significant efforts of social activism.

While the connection between grievances and social movement participation is one of the debates in social movement theory (see Opp, 1988), some argue that social movements can function without collective grievances. Johnston (1980) describes what he calls the marketed social movement, not based on collective grievances, of which the case of TM is a very successful example and which he uses as an ideal type. He does recognize that the movement has goals, if not collective grievances, such as world peace and universal happiness, which presumably distinguish it from other groups, such as those involved in such activities as aerobics or tennis. The professional sexual misconduct movement, however, has grievances that are not collective in that they vary considerably among the participants. It has its analogy in "public interest" movements that "pursued goals linked to the interests of broad, diffuse, disorganized collectivities" (Jenkins, 1983: 531). Jenkins, in describing the research on this issue, however, points out that the people involved in such movements (the general public or middle-class consumers) would not have become involved without the initiative of policy entrepreneurs. Thus, it is not the absence of grievances that distinguishes the professional sexual misconduct movement from other movements but, rather, the absence of entrepreneurs to mobilize activists. There are no counterparts to celebrities such as Elizabeth Taylor raising money for AIDS or Mavis Leno publicizing the plight of women in Afghanistan under the Taliban, who are increasingly essential for a successful social movement (Meyer and Gamson, 1995). The only spokespeople on behalf of professional sexual misconduct are the "experts" who work in the field (like Gary Schoener and Marie Fortune), who are respected and even loved by those in the movement but who are virtually unknown outside it. In addition, very few feminists and lawyers are working for law reform, as was the case in the rape reform movement or in defense of those women who kill their abusers. Nor are there any policy entrepreneurs whose insider status or political skills enable them to initiate and follow through on political reform efforts (Kingdon, 1995). There are not even any Dr. Kevorkians, whose skills lie in his ability to keep the issue of assisted suicide on the public agenda by his outrageous, media-attracting behavior.

Contrast the professional sexual misconduct movement with the efforts to change the position of the mentally ill in our society, which has been able to interest powerful nonvictims in the problem, despite the fact that the mentally ill as a group have not generally been in a position to become activists because of the nature of their problem. For the most part, activism on the issue of the mentally ill has been by others on their behalf (the landmark case of *Wyatt* v. *Stickney* is a prime example; see Jones and Parlour, 1981). When the National Alliance for the Mentally Ill was first formed, it was primarily an organization of parents of mental patients, whose framing of the problem and strategies for change were not the same as those of patients themselves. Recently, this organization has taken in more of the mentally ill who are sufficiently recovered to form a more powerful alliance to get recognition and funding for their cause (Foderaro, 1995). They have also been able to obtain the help of public figures who have recently come forward to speak of their own psychiatric problems or, more commonly, those of members of their family. This adds the "important public figure" component so far lacking in the professional sexual exploitation movement.

THE GOVERNMENT ROLE (OR LACK THEREOF)

A further mark of the relative failure of the professional sexual misconduct movement is the relative lack of input on the part of governmental authorities at any level. While traditional social movement scholarship saw the state as either an adversary or, at best, a passive actor (Gamson, 1990), more recent work points to the role of the state as an important element of a successful social movement. For example, McCarthy (1994) argues that the movement against drunk driving was able to emerge only as a result of earlier efforts of various authorities. One of the marks of the success of the domestic violence movement has been its ability to enlist government resources in its support at a federal, state, and local level. The culmination of these efforts can be seen in the Violence Against Women Act of 1994, which provided not only significant amounts of money for research and services for victims of domestic violence but also the respectability and visibility that come from being on the government agenda.

In the case of professional sexual misconduct, there are state regulatory bodies whose job is to control the behavior of the professions. While all these organizations have made it clear that sexual behavior between a professional and a patient or client is inappropriate and a matter for their control, for the most part, we have seen that such bodies are reluctant to take strong action. The issue is defined in contrast to many other issues they have to deal with that are seen as "much worse," like medical malpractice, which causes physical, rather than psychological, harm. Legislatures have taken up the issue in some contexts, but here, too, it is seen as a matter of *relative* unimportance, especially in contrast to other issues they see as far more serious. By contrast, all 50 states have in the space of a few years passed antistalking laws. These laws appear to be the result of successful efforts to piggyback on the current credibility of domestic violence as a serious issue. Professional sexual exploitation has not found another major issue on which to piggyback in this way.

Individual bureaucrats share this lack of concern; as we have seen, the police and prosecutors are not much interested in professional sexual misconduct, except in egregious cases. Here the professional sexual misconduct movement can be compared to the efforts to combat sexual harassment in the schools, which confront a similar lack of interest; when schools are suffering from the lack of funds for essential tasks and teachers and pupils are afraid of being killed at school, harassment seems rather tame by comparison.

Drunk driving provides a contrast here, too. McCarthy (1994) shows how the local police and prosecutors participated in "helping the activists to cocreate the victim identity" (157). As we have seen, one can hardly argue that the regulatory agencies that address professional sexual misconduct help the complainants create for themselves a victim identity; many victims argue that the role of the agencies has had quite the opposite effect. Some agencies have attempted to blame the victims or to argue that they are fabricating their claims or in other ways diminish the seriousness of their claim. Thus, rather than having the state actively involved in framing the issue as a serious social problem, the state here is framing it as a relatively unimportant issue.

POTENTIAL MEMBERS: WHERE DO THEY COME FROM AND WHAT DO THEY DO?

Implicit in resource mobilization for social movements is the idea that there are specific sources from which activists can be recruited, especially preexisting group organizations (see Jenkins, 1983). In the case of professional sexual misconduct, we have seen that there were no such organizations but, instead, groups that were set up to deal specifically with the issue. As we have seen, even many of the members of these groups are unwilling or unable to move into activism. The groups have remained small and unknown outside the members who use them directly. There is a tremendous need for confidentiality felt by many who have been exploited professionally that limits the lines of communication necessary to maximize the benefits of collective action. It also provides a further reason many victims are unwilling to come out in public and engage in collective action. One of the essential elements of protest is that it has sustained access to arenas of public discourse, which is another indication of the inability of the professional sexual misconduct movement to acquire the necessary public recognition for success.

A further characteristic of this movement that minimizes its success is that the lion's share of those involved in the movement are also victims of the problem. Even among those relatively few professionals who interest themselves in the problem, many of them have also been sexually exploited by professionals, often during their training. Of those who are not themselves victims, most of them are in some way directly involved in the problem and may have an interest different from the goal of social change. Lawyers who work in this area benefit in direct ways from its recognition in cases they can bring; therapists have a direct interest in the victimized patients whom they see as well as an interest in the reputation of their profession. Thus far, the movement has not attracted individuals and groups of people who are activists because they see it as an important social problem. This is another way in which it can be distinguished from the anti-drunk driving movement, which, as Weed (1990) shows, attracts many "nonvictims" who have not themselves been harmed, directly or indirectly, by a drunk driver but who see this as an important social issue. For these people, mostly middle-class women who are also active in other causes, this is a respectable cause in which innocent victims suffer as the result of the wrongdoing of others. The issue is not so clear-cut in the case of professional sexual misconduct; the victims are not seen as so innocent, and the offenders are not yet universally defined as evil. Often, the situation is the reverse: the victim is perceived as consenting or crazy, and the widely respected professional is perceived as the subject of an unfair smear campaign.

Eyerman and Jamison (1991) point out that American social movements are "often, if not always two movements in one" (37). What they mean is that a social movement has a local, activist part and the part with the established organizations with lawyers and lobbyists in Washington. The professional sexual misconduct movement is really only the first part. Just as it has no policy entrepreneurs working for the cause, so, too, it has no lobbyists in Washington or anywhere else. The lawyers mentioned earlier are practitioners in cases that benefit individuals rather than lobbyists for change in general. In some states, lobbyists were hired to help push the criminal legislation through the legislature; they served, however, only for that one issue. In addition, there are relatively few local groups from which to launch collective action. As Jenkins (1983) points out, "The mobilization potential of a group is largely determined by the degree of preexisting group organization" (538). The professional sexual misconduct movement suffers from the fact that it began without preexisting organizations from which it could draw members but instead had to start the process from scratch with groups set up especially for the purpose of combating this problem. Nor have any of the preexisting groups that might be relevant (e.g., the women's movement) branched out to take on the issue of professional sexual misconduct as they did with rape reform and domestic violence (Schechter, 1982; Dobash and Dobash, 1992). The closest thing to a parallel organization is the rape crisis centers, some of which have taken up the issue, albeit as a secondary concern.

"Status movements take action about 'other people's business' because that business often poses a threat to how the mobilizing group defines itself" (Johnson et al., 1994: 23). One can argue that professional sexual misconduct does not pose a sufficient threat to the various potential mobilizing groups (feminists, medical consumers, and even religious groups). McCarthy (1994) points out that "a frame must resonate with the experience of a collectivity and be accessible with its mix of crosscutting identities" (134). Relatively few people, however, appear to see themselves as potential patients or clients in the mental health setting, and many members of religious congregations see clergy abuse as something that happens to children and in other denominations. So the problem of professional sexual misconduct remains "other people's business" to be defined only by those few who are directly threatened by it. This difficulty is compounded by the various different ways it can be framed. If it is framed as a feminist issue, then it is definitely "other people's business" to those who frame it differently, as, for example, a medical/professional issue or a religious issue. The same, of course, is true in reverse.

Contrast this lack of threat to the issue of campus sexual assault (Bohmer and Parrot, 1993). This problem has other constituencies in ways that professional sexual misconduct does not. These constituencies see it as a threat to themselves and therefore worthy of action. First, many young women have not themselves been assaulted but see campus sexual assault as a threat to their self-definition, that is, as potential victims, vulnerable, unequal, and unprotected. Some male students also see the issue as a threat to their self-definition, in this case as predatory monsters, rapists, and abusers of power.

The difference is highlighted by another characteristic that contrasts professional sexual misconduct with campus sexual assault: the former is a very diffuse movement, while the latter is not. Lofland (1969) described the "youth ghetto" in which large concentrations of young people around college campuses increase the likelihood of a variety of potential movements. Thus, one of the current movements occupying the attention of college students is to highlight and deal with the problem of campus sexual assault and rape in general. The annual Take Back the Night marches in campus communities are now a standard part of this movement. Some research has been conducted on other groups that have formed from those who are geographically connected; the best example is that of environmental hazards located in or near a community, like Woburn, Massachusetts (see Harr, 1995), or Three Mile Island. By contrast, the potential members of the professional sexual misconduct movement are scattered all over the country, which exacerbates mobilization problems. As Mueller (1992) points out, "[F]ace-to-face interaction is the social setting from which meanings critical to the interpretation of collective identities, grievances, and opportunities are created, interpreted and transformed" (10). Jenkins (1983) addresses this issue when he says of the younger wing of the women's movement: "Despite rhetorical commitments to institutional change, appropriate actions were organizationally blocked by the decentralized structures" (541). It is for this reason that the conferences, meetings, and support groups described in previous chapters are so essential and why the fact that they are relatively rare and sometimes not well attended has serious ramifications for the movement's success.

WHO BENEFITS FROM ACTIVISM?

Survivors of professional sexual exploitation also have a problem raised by the rational actor model for mobilization for collective action (see Friedman and McAdam, 1992). Given that so many of the members of the social movement have themselves been victims of the behavior they are trying to control, the benefits are, by definition, for others, not for themselves. Thus, a rational actor model has to allow for a cost calculus in which members are willing to participate in collective action primarily for indirect benefit. In light of this and the negative psychological effects of such victimization, it is actually remarkable that *anyone* gets involved in the movement! Benefits are more or less indirect depending on the nature of the activism; for those involved in finding and prosecuting or suing their perpetrator, the benefit is more direct than for those working, for example, to change the law so that subsequent perpetrators will be punished. But social change is more likely to take place as a result of the latter rather than the former. Many of the efforts described earlier have addressed individual, rather than group, benefits, which severely limits the potential social change in the movement. Framing is relevant here, too; many of the victims who sue their perpetrators and do benefit directly often describe the benefits in terms of how they will help others rather than themselves (see also Bohmer and Parrot, 1993, for similar goals on the part of campus sexual assault victims). So, too, do those who complain to regulatory agencies. Thus, only by defining benefits in an indirect way can the rational actor model be made to fit this case.

CONCLUSION

Feminists have critiqued resource mobilization theory for its assumption of the separation of public life from personal life (Gagne, 1998). New social movement theory allows for the examination of activism in all aspects of life, including the personal. Verta Taylor (1996) argues that this broader approach makes possible an analysis of the "significant social and cultural transformations that shaped the character of social movements in the 1980s" (89). Even within this broader frame of analysis, however, when the movement to publicize and change professional sexual exploitation is compared to other new social movements, it has not been very successful. We have seen the ways in which the nature of the problem mitigates against movement success in a variety of ways.

Comparison with measures of success for the battered women's movement may be instructive here. Both movements primarily involve women victims, and both involve reframing to move the debate from a framework of adult consensual behavior from which any sensible woman would have removed herself, to one of violence or exploitation of an unwilling and powerless victim who could not simply absent herself from the exploitative situation. Both were initially framed as private behavior beyond the scope of public and government intervention. But domestic violence has been more successful in moving beyond that framework than has professional sexual misconduct. Frightening, widely publicized statistics have made the scope of the problem a matter of public awareness both in the criminal justice system and in the wider society. But neither domestic violence nor professional sexual misconduct can boast of a hugely successful slogan like "Friends don't let friends drive drunk" of the movement against drunk driving. As in the case of professional sexual misconduct, many people still adhere to the earlier framework of battering as private behavior from which a woman is responsible for removing herself.

Nevertheless, there have been widespread changes in the criminal law relating to domestic violence and the way it is administered (Dobash and Dobash, 1992; Schechter, 1982). A number of well-publicized civil and criminal lawsuits have increased awareness as well as changing the law in significant ways. Specialist lawyers and university law clinics have become involved in acting on behalf of victims of domestic violence, especially those who kill their abusers (Gagne, 1998). Governments at all levels have been willing to provide funding and other support for a number of aspects of the problem, ranging from shelters, to social service agencies, to victim advocacy, to research (Crowell and Burgess, 1996).

This chapter has shown some of the reasons for the discrepancy in the two social movements. Some of the reasons may be time-based and may change in the future, while others appear to be inherent in the nature of the problem itself. It has also shown some of the reasons professional sexual misconduct has been less than successful as a social movement generally and when compared to a variety of other social movements.

NOTE

1. There is now a countermovement to return to the fault-based laws, which were changed so effectively in the 1970s.

—10—

WHERE TO NOW?

Women who seek help from professionals are vulnerable by virtue of that need for help. Despite the rhetoric that victims are just like anyone else, researchers have found that a high proportion of them fall into particular vulnerable groups. Quadrio (1994) argues that four groups of women are vulnerable to therapist abuse: "those who have experienced childhood physical or sexual abuse; those who have experienced neglect; the childhood caretakers or other paternified children; and those with a devalued 'masculine' self" (19). Luepker (1999) found that 60 percent of the women in her study who were the subjects of professional sexual misconduct by various professionals had previously experienced unwanted sexual touching by an adult or older child, and 64 percent had previously been the recipient of physical abuse. These rates may be higher because both researchers were dealing with clinical populations, but nevertheless, all evidence suggests that the risk is higher for vulnerable women.

Men who sexually exploit their patients or clients know that these people are vulnerable, not just because the men know of the prior abuse but because they sense a vulnerability that makes the women suitable targets for abuse (Wohlberg, 1993).

When therapists are caught and accused of sexual misconduct, they exhibit a variety of responses. Some of them justify their actions in ways similar to those they first used to justify the behavior to their patients, generally in terms of the benefits to the patient. Others continue to deny the behavior, usually arguing that the woman is hysterical and a liar. Jules Masserman, even after hearings by the board and an extended civil trial in which it was shown that he drugged his patients before having sex with them, continued to maintain his innocence: "I never did anything unethical with any patient" (Noel with Watterson, 1992: 319). Still others admit their misconduct and justify it in terms of their personal problems, while others offer no justification at all (Pogrebin et al., 1992).

Whatever their explanations, the professionals' behavior is made possible by the vulnerability of the patient or client and the power of the professional. In therapeutic relationships the power is inherent in the relationship itself, described as transference in the professional literature. As Gabbard and Nadelson (1995) put it, in describing the psychological state of the patient because of the clinical relationship: "Patients rapidly develop feelings toward their physicians that have been called 'transference.' The physician can thus be viewed as an all-knowing parent, and a great deal of power is turned over to the physician by the patient" (144–47).

Thus, the social roles of the person in need of help and the person administering that help exacerbate the power imbalance, especially when the patient or client is female. In fact, the fatherly professional responding to the needs of the childlike patient or client is the archetypical patriarchal relationship. As we have seen, these social roles color the adjudication of complaints. As long as those hearing complaints represent the father and those complaining represent the child (usually female), the complainant is less likely to be believed than the fatherly professional.

Thus, a combination of vulnerability on the part of the patient or client and the abuse of the very great power residing in the professional seems to be the recipe for professional sexual misconduct. But, of course, most professionals do not abuse their patients. Little is known about why some professionals do so and continue to do so, in the face of the clear ethical prohibitions in many professions and some publicity of the issue in the professional and general media. We have seen, however, that even though there has been some publicity about the issue, many aspects of the problem are not given more than sporadic coverage, which might make it easier for the abusing professional to deny the existence of the prohibitions.

Schoener (19 May 1998) argues that education is a crucial element in the prevention of sexual exploitation in the professional relationship. He remains concerned about how little real education is currently being undertaken in the training of professionals, even after the ethical issue has been clear for so long. He sees the need for education as part of a multipronged approach, which is best exemplified by his home state of Minnesota. He believes that there has been a genuine decline in the incidence of professional sexual misconduct in Minnesota, though, of course, this is hard to document. He points out that the Walk-In Counselling Center has not been able to get together a therapy group for survivors of professional sexual misconduct for well over a year. In addition, there have been fewer cases tried recently both in court and by the relevant boards. He believes that some abusing professionals have left the state, while others have reported that they were scared off for fear of being caught (Schoener, 21 October 1996).

Schoener's suggested multipronged approach contains the following elements:

1. *A criminal statute.* As we have seen, Minnesota's statute, the second in the nation, was passed in 1985 and was the result of a task force that held hearings around the state, which generated significant publicity.

2. *A civil statute.* This has several important elements. First, as we have seen in Chapter 6, it has the benefit of making it easier for a plaintiff to sue in civil court. The Minnesota statute defines "psychotherapist" broadly, so that it also includes pastoral counselors as well as unlicensed therapists. It provides for a suit based on posttermination sex. It requires employers to take steps to prevent and report sexual contact between therapists/employees and patients (Bisbing et al., 1995: 223). This means that employers are now careful to conduct background checks on potential employees in order to comply with the statute and to limit their liability. The civil statute in Minnesota requires a subsequent therapist who knows or suspects prior therapist abuse to report that abuse, including the name of the suspected abuser. The statute also requires that informational brochures be made available.

3. *Improvement in the response of licensing authorities.* Minnesota has "beefed up" its regulatory actions against suspected sexually abusing professionals (Schoener, 21 October 1996). This not only serves to provide some remedy to the victims but also sends a message to other potential abusers.

4. *Education and information.* The very presence of the only specialized clinic for victims of professional sexual misconduct, the Walk-In Counselling Center in Minneapolis, makes a great difference here. Schoener and his colleagues are engaged in an ongoing effort of education and public awareness. Other Minnesota institutions, including several churches, are also actively involved in education as well as training of their clergy members.

Combined, this package seems to have had an effect on the incidence of professional sexual misconduct in the state. Schoener is quick to point out that in order to reduce the incidence of professional sexual misconduct, a state needs to address the problem with a number of different measures, such as those described. As we have seen, a number of other states have taken some steps, but none have Minnesota's comprehensive approach.

While the problem of professional sexual misconduct does not affect only women, it does, however, affect mostly women. Part of the reason the problem has not received as much attention as it deserves has to do with that fact. Despite gains made in other issues affecting women, like domestic violence and rape, it nevertheless remains true that "men's issues" are seen as more important and receive more attention than do "women's issues." Not only are women generally involved in this issue, but they are also much more involved in help-seeking behavior than are men. In addition, the problem involves mental health issues, another taboo subject in which sufferers are seen as weak and not suitably self-reliant. All these aspects of the problem combine to keep professional sexual misconduct on the back burner. In the meantime, the issue remains a major problem for most of those who are exploited by a professional they have trusted. Despite the many studies of incidence and outcome, we still know relatively little about exactly how many people are exploited sexually by professionals or how seriously they suffer. Those who do come to the attention of subsequent treating professionals are likely to be those who have suffered more. The patients and clients who were able to put the experience behind them are unlikely to appear in any of the statistics or to come forward in response to my requests for interviews. I have met survivors who are still reliving their experiences 30 years later. Others have committed suicide as a result of the damage caused by their exploitation at a very vulnerable time.

SO, HOW FAR HAVE WE COME, AND WHAT OF THE FUTURE?

Lest this book end on too pessimistic a note, the final section summarizes the achievements of the efforts for public recognition and change in professional sexual misconduct. It also looks to the future to see where the movement is headed.

As late as the 1970s, some therapists were officially arguing that therapist–patient sex could be therapeutic. One sign of progress is that no one argues that now. On the contrary, all the professional associations, except legal associations, have very clearly stated that professional–client sex is unethical and prohibited behavior by members. Most licensing boards have similarly specific injunctions. Not only is the behavior prohibited, but in some cases the exact nature of the behavior is described, including when therapy begins and ends for the purpose of this prohibition.

While there is a very long way to go, licensing boards have begun to take the problem seriously and to hear more claims of professional sexual misconduct. Even though we have seen that many decisions by the licensing boards fall short of loss of license, they are all invasive and require the professional to defend himself against the accusations, with consequent damage to his professional standing and financial well-being. Even the role of ethics boards has had some effect, if only in making it more difficult for a professional with an ethical violation to obtain insurance or an affiliation with a health maintenance organization.

In addition, there have been a number of well-publicized court cases, especially in the case of the clergy. The Catholic Church has been most reluctant to address the problem openly, despite having been alerted to its pervasiveness many years ago. The court defeats may succeed in doing what years of other kinds of pressure have failed to do: have the clergy address the problem immediately instead of transferring the priest from one parish to another after he has been "cured" at one of the church's centers. By contrast, some other churches have been in the forefront in addressing the issue. They have made valiant efforts to confront the problem head on and have produced model education and training programs.

Court victories have a broad impact for many people. Hearing of substantial jury verdicts paid to victims of professional sexual abuse provides credibility to the movement that other victories may not. In our society, nothing seems to clear the mind like the award of a large sum to an innocent plaintiff. Even those whose behavior may not be changed by moral imperatives may be deterred by the fear of a large money verdict against them for such behavior.

We have also seen the movement for criminal legislation to outlaw therapist–patient sex. Again, the impact of this legislation has been limited, but it has had some effect in publicizing the behavior. Many people do not want to frame this as a criminal issue; this does not mean, however, that they do not believe it is wrong and should not be punished in some way. The criminal legislation has the function of providing a benchmark against which to measure the appropriate punishment—if not jail, then loss of license or some other negative outcome.

Some states have acted in various ways to prevent professional sexual exploitation. We discussed Minnesota, but other states have also made efforts to take the problem seriously. For example, Maryland had a task force to examine the issue and followed that with recommendations for statutory changes that the task force believed were both politically realistic and would have a significant impact on the problem. Unlike other states, one piece of legislation recently passed requires regulatory boards to report annual statistics of the number and disposition of sexual misconduct complaints and also to include in their regulations a specific definition of sexual misconduct (Senate Bill 495, March 1998). Other states have put in place some of the pieces of the Minnesota approach, though none have adopted the entire package.

One important issue addressed by a number of states is consumer education. We have seen how difficult it is for consumers, first, to know that the behavior was unethical and, second, to know what choices they have if they want to take action. Some states have mandated the provision of consumer brochures in various places; how accessible they are to those who have been exploited is not clear. Nevertheless, it represents an important step in consumer education, especially as many victims of professional sexual misconduct do not know that it is unethical or, in some states, even illegal.

Consumer education is part of a broader process of education that includes everyone who is involved in the issue. Schoener (19 May 1998) argues that education of the professions is an essential element of a prevention program for professional sexual misconduct. We have seen that most of those professionals who exploit their patients or clients sexually are also involved in other boundary violations. Thus, education about the nature of these boundary violations and how to address them before they develop into sexual misconduct is an essential element of professional education. At the moment this education is rather sporadically available and does not go nearly far enough to reach all the professionals (Schoener, 19 May 1998).

With its multipronged approach, Minnesota has shown that it is possible to reduce the incidence of professional sexual misconduct, although it is difficult to provide empirical evidence to support this conclusion. It is even more difficult to provide evidence of changes in the incidence of professional sexual misconduct in other parts of the country. The Minnesota model is based on a combination of publicity, education, deterrence, and sure punishment. Whether the various efforts made by Minnesota or any other state do serve as a deterrent for professional sexual abuse is difficult to determine empirically. Scholars have enough difficulty assessing the value and effectiveness of deterrence in less diffuse situations, so it is impossible to make any forceful statements about the value of deterrence in this case. It does seem that deterrence can work for at least some potential offenders. Those who were unaware of the issue and the damage it could cause may now know enough to be deterred, as may those who have learned about the financial and career risks involved. Younger people seem to be less at risk, which bodes well for the future (Dehlendorf and Wolfe, 1997). There are, nevertheless, a few people who "just don't get it" and who are not affected by any amount of publicity and continue because they are so arrogant or such predators that deterrence is irrelevant.

As for the future, I predict more of the same. I do not believe that the professional sexual misconduct movement will ever be widely recognized and well-financed. I do, however, believe that the steps that have been taken in the last decade or two will continue. Gradually, the movement will gain acceptability among those for whom it is central, the professionals themselves. Just as, for example, rape crisis centers seemed so radical 25 years ago but are now commonplace and unquestioned recipients of government funding, so, perhaps, will professional sexual misconduct be accepted without question as unethical and beyond the pale. Professionals who engage in sexual misconduct may also come to be shunned by their colleagues, instead of supported, as so many of them still are.

More specifically, I believe that there will be more by way of consumer education. This generation no longer relies on the word of the kindly, paternal doctor for medical information but, instead, looks to the Internet and other sources for information. There is already a Web site that provides some information to consumers; no doubt available information will increase as use of the Web continues to increase.

Technology may also provide the remedy for some of the gaps we have seen in the system, for example, connections among the various remedies for those who have been exploited sexually by professionals. Technology will continue to make the transfer of information between one state authority and another easier, which will make it more difficult for a professional found guilty of professional sexual misconduct in one state to move his practice elsewhere. This is already happening in the medical field and will continue there and in other professions.

I am less optimistic about the way licensing boards handle their cases. As long as they are underfunded, and the incidence is not significantly reduced, backlogs that ensure that cases take a very long time to process will continue. Improvement in the follow-up of professionals who have been required to undertake some training or therapy will also not take place until the boards obtain increased resources and more education about the nature of appropriate follow-up. So far, they do not seem very willing to learn. But maybe the drip, drip, drip approach will affect licensing boards, too. If the incidence can be reduced by increased publicity and education, and if younger professionals continue to exhibit lower rates of sexual misconduct, boards may be able to deal with the cases they have more effectively.

Finally, more women may be aware of the possibility of professional sexual misconduct *before* they enter a professional relationship. These women may be less likely to accept the framing offered by professionals, especially those who argue that the relationship is for the women's own good. Maybe fewer professionals will take advantage of those patients and clients who by virtue of their condition are in no position to take the responsibility of resisting the advances of those in power over them.

REFERENCES

Acker, Alex J. "Alex's Story." *Breach of Trust: Sexual Exploitation by Health Care Professionals and Clergy.* Ed. John C. Gonsiorek. Thousand Oaks, CA: Sage, 1995. 45–48.

Alexander, Joan. Personal interview. 2 December 1993a.

———. "Texas Is Waking Up to the Horrors Inflicted by Psychological Predators." *Houston Chronicle* 3 October 1993b: 1F.

Allen, Martha Sawyer. "Clergy Abuse Suit Dismissed; Story Was Made Up, Roach Says." *Star Tribune* 26 June 1993: 1A, 11A.

American Psychiatric Association. *Resource Document: Legal Sanctions for Mental Health Professional–Patient Sex.* Washington, DC: American Psychiatric Association, 1993.

Anderson, Jeffrey. "How to Find Healing and Hold Church Leaders Accountable Employing a Legal Strategy." First International SNAP Conference, Washington, DC, 9 November 1996.

Andrews, Arlene Bowers. *Victimization and Survivor Services. A Guide to Victim Assistance.* New York: Springer, 1992.

Angier, Natalie. "In the History of Gynecology, a Surprising Chapter 'Hydro-Massage.'" *New York Times* 23 February 1999: 5D.

Athena. Personal communication. 4 June 1999.

Bandura, Albert. *Aggression: A Social Learning Analysis.* Englewood Cliffs, NJ: Prentice-Hall, 1973.

Barbara. Personal interview. 23 October 1998.

Barron, N., L. I. Eakins, and R. Wollert. "Fat Group: A Snap-Launched Self-Help Group." *Human Organization* 43.1 (1984): 44–49.

Bass, Alison. "Therapist Accused of Sex Abuse of Clients." *Boston Globe* 5 March 1989: 1.

Bass, Alison, and Judy Foreman. "Therapist Accused of Sex Abuse Resigns License." *Boston Globe* 4 April 1989: 17–18.

Bayles, Michael D. "Professional Power and Self-Regulation." *Business and Professional Ethics Journal* 5.2 (1986): 26–46.

Bender, Leslie. "An Overview of the Feminist Tort Scholarship." *Cornell Law Review* 78 (1993): 575–96.

Benowitz, Mindy. "Sexual Exploitation of Female Clients by Female Therapists." Ph.D. diss., University of Minnesota, 1991.

Berger, Ronald J., Patricia Searles, and W. Lawrence Neuman. "The Dimensions of Rape Reform Legislation." *Law and Society Review* 22 (1988): 329–57.

Berry, Jason. *Lead Us Not into Temptation.* New York: Doubleday, 1992.

Best, Joel. *Threatened Children.* Chicago: University of Chicago Press, 1990.

———. *Images of Issues.* New York: Aldine de Gruyter, 1989.

Bisbing, Steven B., Linda Mabus Jorgenson, and Pamela K. Sutherland. *Sexual Abuse by Professionals: A Legal Guide Supplement.* Charlottesville, VA: Michie, 1999.

———. *Sexual Abuse by Professionals: A Legal Guide. Cumulative Supplement.* Charlottesville, VA: Michie, 1998.

———. *Sexual Abuse by Professionals: A Legal Guide Supplement.* Charlottesville, VA: Michie, 1997.

———. *Sexual Abuse by Professionals: A Legal Guide.* Charlottesville, VA: Michie, 1995.

Blaine, Barbara. Presentation at the First International SNAP Conference, Washington, DC, 8 November 1996.

Board of Registration in Medicine (Mass.) v. *Joel Feigen, M.D.* Docket RM 90–1304, 75–77 (1/27/92).

Bohmer, Carol. "Failure and Success in Self-Help Groups for Victims of Professional Sexual Exploitation." *Journal of Community Psychology* 23 (1995a): 190–9.

———. "Regulating Professional Sexual Misconduct: Does It Work and How Can You Tell?" Paper presented at the Law and Society Meetings, Toronto, Canada. 1–4 June 1995b.

———. "Victims Who Fight Back: Claiming in Cases of Professional Sexual Exploitation." *Justice System Journal* 16.3 (1994): 73–92.

———. "Acquaintance Rape and the Law." *Acquaintance Rape: The Hidden Crime.* Eds. Andrea Parrot and Laurie Bechhofer. New York: John Wiley & Sons Inc., 1991. 317–33.

Bohmer, Carol, and Andrea Parrot. *Sexual Assault on Campus: The Problem and the Solution.* New York: Lexington Press, 1993.

Borkman, T. J. "Experiential Professional and Lay Frames of Reference." *Working with Self-Help.* Ed. T. Powell. Silver Spring, MD: National Association of Social Workers, 1990. 3–30.

Bouhoutsos, Jacqueline, et al. "Sexual Intimacy between Therapists and Patients." *Professional Psychology* 14 (1983): 185–96.

Bourque, Linda. *Defining Rape.* Durham, NC: Duke University Press, 1989.

Brint, Steven. *In an Age of Experts.* Princeton, NJ: Princeton University Press, 1994.

Broken Boundaries: Sexual Exploitation in the Professional-Client Relationship. Baltimore: Maryland Department of Health and Mental Hygiene, 1999.

Brown, Laura S. "Coping with 'Mind-Rape': Non-Sexual Abuse in Therapy." Paper presented at It's Never O.K. Conference, Toronto, Canada, 1994a.

———. Personal interview. 15 October 1994b.

Bunes, Heidi E. Personal communication. 7 July 1994.

Butler, Sandra. "Breaking and Entering: When Trust Is Shattered." Paper presented to It's Never O.K. Conference, Toronto, Canada, 1994.

Butterfield, Fox. "Diocese Reaches Settlement with 68 Who Accuse Priest of Sexual Abuse." *New York Times* 4 December 1992a: 8A.

———. "Panel Orders a Hearing in Bizarre Harvard Case." *New York Times* 31 March 1992b.

C. D. Personal communication. 5 June 1999.

Campbell, Vicki. Personal communication. 6 March 1999.

Carol. Personal interview. 24 June 1993.

Chesler, Phyllis. *Women and Madness*. New York: Avon Books, 1972.

Christie, Nils. "The Ideal Victim." *From Crime Policy to Victim Policy*. Ed. Ezzat A. Fattah. New York: St. Martin's Press, 1986. 17–39.

Cindy. Personal interview. 7 November 1993.

Clark, Robert C. "Why Does Health Care Regulation Fail?" *Maryland Law Review* 41.1 (1981): 1–29.

Clarke, Alicia J., and Jeffrey E. Barnett. "Report on SPPA's Ethics Committees: A 1997–98 Comprehensive Survey of Current Roles and Practices." Paper presented to the 106th Annual Conference of the American Psychological Association, August 1998.

———. "Investigation Practices of State Psychological Associations' Ethics Committees." N.d.

Clohessy, David. Personal interview. 28 March and 19 September 1995.

Cole, Susan. "The Yawn Syndrome." Paper presented at It's Never O.K. Conference, Toronto, Canada, 1994.

Collison, M. "A Berkeley Scholar Clashes with Feminists over Validity of Their Research on Date Rape." *Chronicle of Higher Education* 26 February 1992: 29A.

Constantinides, Criton A. "Note: Professional Ethics Codes in Court: Redefining the Social Contract between the Public and the Professions." *Georgia Law Review* 25 (1991): 1327–73.

Crews, Frederick. "Victims of Repressed Memory." *The New York Review of Books* 41.19 (1994): 54–60 and 41.20 (1994): 49–58.

Crichton, Michael. *Disclosure*. New York: A. A. Knopf, 1994.

Crossing the Boundaries: The Report of the Committee on Physician Sexual Misconduct. Vancouver, Canada: College of Physicians and Surgeons of British Columbia, 1992.

Crowe, Donald. Personal interview. 10 March 1999.

———. "Letter to the Los Angeles Psychological Society Newsletter." *Los Angeles Psychological Society Newsletter* (June 1998): 3.

Crowell, Nancy A., and Ann W. Burgess. *Understanding Violence against Women*. Washington, DC: National Academy Press, 1996.

Cudahy, V. Personal interview. 27 October 1993.

D'Addario, Linda. *Sexual Relationships between Female Clients and Male Therapists*. San Diego: California School of Professional Psychology, 1977.

Dahlberg, Clay. "Sexual Contact between Client and Therapist." *Contemporary Psychoanalysis* 6 (1970): 1007–124.

Daniels, Stephen, Jerry Van Hoy, and Joanne Martin. "Clouds and Silver Linings: The Response of Plaintiffs' Lawyers to Tort Reform." Paper presented to the Law and Society Meetings, Chicago, 27–30 May 1999.

Davidson, Virginia. "Psychiatry's Problem with No Name: Therapist–Patient Sex." *The American Journal of Psychoanalysis* 37.1 (1977): 43–50.

Dehlendorf, Christine E., and Sidney M. Wolfe. "Physicians Disciplined for Sex-Related Offenses." Washington, DC: Public Citizen Health Research Group, 1997.

Demarest, Sylvia (Attorney for plaintiffs in case against Diocese of Dallas). Personal interview. 15 February 1999; 8 November 1997.

Dempsey, Laurel. "Progress Report: Mandatory Reporting of Sexual Abuse." *Members' Dialogue* (November 1994): 23.

Department of Business and Professional Regulation v. *Price*. 1994. Final Order No. BPR-94-00001614.

Devlin, Kathy. Personal interview. 7 February 1999.

Dingwall, Robert, and Philip Lewis. *The Sociology of the Professions*. London: Macmillan, 1983.

Disch, Estelle, and Janet W. Wohlberg. "The Boston Experience: Responding to Sexual Abuse by Professionals." *Breach of Trust: Sexual Exploitation by Health Care Professionals and Clergy*. Ed. John C. Gonsiorek. Thousand Oaks, CA: Sage, 1995. 57–74.

Dobash, R. Emerson, and Russell P. Dobash. *Women, Violence and Social Change*. New York: Routledge, 1992.

Dolan, Andrew K., and Nicole D. Urban. "The Determinants of the Effectiveness of Medical Disciplinary Boards: 1960–1977." *Law and Human Behavior* 7.2/3 (1983): 203–17.

Doro, Carol. Personal interview. 24 June 1993.

Downs, Anthony. "Up and Down with Ecology: The Issue Attention Cycle." *Public Interest* 28 (1972): 38–50.

Durkin, Tom. "Framing the Choice to Sue: Victim Cognitions and Claims." *American Bar Foundation*. Working paper #9119, 1991.

Economous, Tom. "The Shamefulness of Cardinal Roger Mahony and the Los Angeles Diocese." *Missing Link* 7.1 (1999): 1.

———. Personal interview. 8 November 1997.

———. "Bishops Find 'Loopholes' in Battle Against Clergy Sexual Abuse." *Missing Link* 4.1 (1996): 1.

———. Personal interview. 20 September 1995.

Elazar, Daniel J. *American Federalism: A View from the States*. New York: Harper and Row, 1984.

Elias, Robert. *The Politics of Victimization: Victims, Victimology and Human Rights*. New York: Oxford University Press, 1986.

Erickson, Mary (Minnesota Board of Medical Practice). Personal interview. 6 May 1998.

Erickson, Robert S., Gerald C. Wright, and John P. McIver. *Statehouse Democracy: Public Opinion and Policy in the American States*. New York: Cambridge University Press, 1993.

Erlich, Susan, and Ruth King. "Feminist Meanings and the (De)politicization of the Lexicon." *Language and Society* 23 (1994): 59–76.

Estrich, Susan. *Real Rape*. Cambridge: Harvard University Press, 1987.

"Ex-Priest Gets Jail in Sex Case." *New York Times* 29 January 1993: 9A.

"Ex-Priest Goes to Prison for Sex Crimes in the 1960's." *New York Times* 7 December 1993: 7A.

Eyerman, Ron, and Andrew Jamison. *Social Movements: A Cognitive Approach.* University Park: Pennsylvania State University Press, 1991.

FBI. *Uniform Crime Reports.* Washington, DC: U.S. Department of Justice, 1982.

Felstiner, William, Richard Abel, and Austin Sarat. "The Emergence and Transformation of Disputes: Naming, Blaming, Claiming. . . ." *Law and Society Journal* 15 (1981): 631–54.

Firestone, Marvin H., and Robert I. Simon. "Intimacy versus Advocacy: Attorney–Client Sex." *Tort and Insurance Law Journal* 27.4 (1992): 679–91.

Firsten, Terri. "Opening Remarks." Paper presented at It's Never OK Conference, Toronto, Canada, 14 October 1994.

Fisher, Elizabeth. Personal interview. 16 May 1993.

Fiske, Susan T., and Shelley E. Taylor. *Social Cognition.* Reading, MA: Addison-Wesley, 1983.

Fitzpatrick, Frank. *Survivor Activist.* 4.3 (1996): 6.

———. "Frank Fitzpatrick's Story." *Survivor Connections Introductory Package.* Cranston, RI: Survivor Connections, n.d. 1.

———. Personal interview. 5 September 1995.

Fitzpatrick, Sara. Personal interview. 5 September 1995, 3 June 1994.

Foderaro, Lisa W. "Mentally Ill Gaining New Rights with the Ill as Their Own Lobby." *New York Times* 14 October 1995: 1A.

Ford, David A. "Prosecution as a Victim Power Resource: A Note on Empowering Women in Violent Conjugal Relationships." *Law and Society Review* 25.2 (1991): 313–34.

Fortune, Marie M. "How Survivors Are Healing and How Church Leaders Are Responding with an Emphasis on Those Abused by Adults." Paper presented to the First International SNAP Conference, Washington, DC, 8–10 November, 1996.

———. "Is Nothing Sacred: When Sex Invades the Pastoral Relationship." *Breach of Trust: Sexual Exploitation by Health Care Professionals and Clergy.* Ed. John C. Gonsiorek. Thousand Oaks, CA: Sage, 1995. 29–40.

———. *Is Nothing Sacred?* New York: Harper and Row, 1989.

France, Jane. Personal inteview. 24 January 1996.

Freeman, Lucy, and Julie Roy. *Betrayal.* New York: Stein and Day, 1976.

Freud, Sigmund. "Introductory Lectures in Psychoanalysis." *The Standard Edition of the Complete Psychological Works of Sigmund Freud.* Vol. 16. Ed. J. Strachey. London: Hogarth Press, 1958.

Friedman, Debra, and Doug McAdam. "Collective Identity and Activism: Networks, Choices, and the Life of a Social Movement." *Frontiers in Social Movement Theory.* Ed. Aldon D. Morris and Carol McClurg Mueller. New Haven, CT: Yale University Press, 1992. 156–73.

Friedman, Joel, and Marcia Mobilia Boumil. *Betrayal of Trust.* Westport, CT: Praeger, 1995.

Friedson, Eliot. *Professional Powers.* Chicago: University of Chicago Press, 1986.

Gabbard, Glen O. "Psychotherapists Who Transgress Sexual Boundaries with Patients." *Breach of Trust: Sexual Exploitation by Health Care Professionals and Clergy.* Ed. John C. Gonsiorek. Thousand Oaks, CA: Sage, 1995.

Gabbard, Glen O., and Carol Nadelson. "Professional Boundaries in the Physician–Patient Relationship." *Journal of the American Medical Association* 273.18 (1995): 1445–49.

Gagne, Patricia. *Battered Women's Justice*. New York: Twayne, 1998.

Gamson, William. *The Strategy of Social Protest*. Belmont, CA: Wadsworth, 1990.

Gardner, Barbara. Personal interview. 7 February 1995.

Gartrell, Nanette, Judith L. Herman, Silvia Olarte, Michael Feldstein, and Russell Localio. "Reporting Practices of Psychiatrists Who Knew of Sexual Misconduct by Colleagues." *American Journal of Orthopsychiatry* 57 (1987): 287–95.

———. "Psychiatrist–Patient Sexual Contact: Results of a National Survey, I: Prevalence." *American Journal of Psychiatry* 143 (1986): 1126–31.

Gentry, Carol. "Abused by the System." *St. Petersburg Times* 26 April 1993.

Geyelin, Milo. "Legal Beat: Churches Find Themselves Hit by More Suits." *Wall Street Journal* 12 November 1992: 1B, 16B.

Glick, Henry R. *The Right to Die: Policy Innovation and Its Consequences*. New York: Columbia University Press, 1992.

Godstein, Laurie. "Hare Krishna Movement Details Past Abuse at Its Boarding Schools." *New Tork Times* 9 October 1998: 1A, 14A.

Gonsiorek, John C., ed. *Breach of Trust: Sexual Exploitation by Health Care Professionals and Clergy*. Thousand Oaks, CA: Sage, 1995.

Gonsiorek, John C., William Bera, and D. LeTourneau. *Male Sexual Abuse: A Trilogy of Intervention Strategies*. Thousand Oaks, CA: Sage, 1994.

Gourley, Kevin. Personal interview. 10 February 1999a.

———. Personal communication. 5 June 1999b.

Greeley, Andrew. *Christian Century* 14 April 1993: 323.

Greenson, Ralph R. *The Technique and Practice of Psychoanalysis*. Vol. 1. New York: International Universities Press, 1967.

Grier, Ruth (Hon. Ontario Minister of Health). Address to It's Never O.K. Conference, Toronto, Canada, 1994.

Gunn, Rita, and Candice Minch. *Sexual Assault: The Dilemma of Disclosure, the Question of Conviction*. Winnipeg, Manitoba: University of Manitoba Press, 1988.

Hall, Terrie. Personal interview. 16 June 1994.

Harr, Jonathan. *A Civil Action*. New York: Random House, 1995.

Harris, E. K. "The Self-Help Approach to Sjögren's Syndrome." *Self-Help Concepts and Applications*. Ed. A. H. Katz, H. L. Hedrick, D. H. Isenberg, L. M. Thompson, T. Goodrich, and A. H. Kutschner. Philadelphia: Charles Press, 1992. 204–13.

Harris v. *Forklift Systems, Inc.* 1993. 114 S. Ct. 367.

Haskin, Gretchen. Personal interview. 12 November 1993.

Herman, Judith L., and Mary R. Harvey. "The False Memory Debate: Social Science or Social Backlash?" *Harvard Mental Health Letter* 9 (1993): 4–6.

Heywood, Carter. "Can Boundaries Betray Us? The Complexity of Ethics in Counselling and Therapy." Paper presented at It's Never O.K. Conference, Toronto, Canada, 1994.

———. *When Boundaries Betray Us: Beyond Illusions of What Is Ethical in Therapy and Life*. New York: Harper, 1993.

Hoffman, J. "Murder Case Damages Faith in Confidentiality of Therapy." *New York Times* 15 June 1994: 1A–13A.

Holmstrom, Lynda Lytle, and Ann Wolbert Burgess. *The Victim of Rape: Institutional Reactions*. New Brunswick, NJ: Transaction, 1983.

Holroyd, Jean C., and Annette M. Brodsky. "Psychologists' Attitudes and Practices regarding Erotic and Nonerotic Physical Contact with Patients." *American Psychologist* 32 (1977): 843–49.

Holstein, James A., and Gale Miller. "Rethinking Victimization: An Interactionist Approach to Victimology." *Symbolic Interaction* 13 (1990): 103–22.

Hux, Katherine P. (Executive Director, Maryland Psychiatric Association). Personal interview. 2 November 1995.

Ibarre, Peter R., and John J. Kitsuse. "Vernacular Constituents of Moral Discourse: An Interactionist Proposal for the Study of Social Problems." *Reconsidering Social Constructionism*. Ed. James A. Holstein and Gale Miller. New York: Aldine de Gruyter, 1993.

In re Gibson. 1985. 369 N.W. 2d 695 (Wis.).

Ingram, H., and D. E. Mann. "Policy Failure: An Issue Deserving Analysis." *Why Policies Succeed or Fail*. Ed. H. Ingram and D. E. Mann. Beverly Hills, CA: Sage, 1980. 11–32.

Isely, Paul J. "The Catholic Church and Child Sexual Abuse: An Historical and Contemporary Examination." Paper presented at First International SNAP Conference, Washington, DC. 8 November 1996.

It's Never O.K.: Third International Conference on Sexual Exploitation by Health Professionals, Psychotherapists and Clergy, Toronto, Canada, 13–15 October 1994.

Jacob, Herbert. *Silent Revolution: The Transformation of Divorce Law in the United States*. Chicago: University of Chicago Press, 1988.

Jan A. Personal communication. 6 June 1999.

Janie. Personal communication. 11 May 1999.

Jehu, Derek. *Patients as Victims*. New York: Wiley, 1994.

Jenkins, J. Craig. "Resource Mobilization Theory and the Study of Social Movements." Ed. Ralph H. Turner and James F. Short. *Annual Review of Sociology* 9 (1983): 527–53.

Jenkins, Philip. *Pedophiles and Priests: Anatomy of a Contemporary Crisis*. New York: Oxford University Press, 1996.

———. "Clergy Sexual Abuse: The Symbolic Politics of a Social Problem." *Images of Issues*. Ed. Joel Best. New York: Aldine de Gruyter, 1995. 105–30.

Jenness, Valerie. "Social Movement Growth, Domain Expansion, and Framing Processes: The Case of Violence against Gays and Lesbians as a Social Problem." *Social Problems* 42.1 (1995): 145–70.

Johnson, Terence J. *Professions and Power*. London: Macmillan, 1972.

Johnston, Hank. "The Marketed Social Movement: A Case Study of the Rapid Growth of TM." *Pacific Sociological Review* 23.3 (1980): 333–54.

Johnston, Hank, and Bert Klandermans. "The Cultural Analysis of Social Movements." *Social Movements and Culture*. Eds. Hank Johnston and Bert Klandermans. Minneapolis: University of Minnesota Press, 1995. 3–24.

Johnston, Hank, Enrique Larana, and Joseph Gusfield. "Identities, Grievances, and New Social Movements." *New Social Movements*. Ed. Hank Johnston, Enrique Larana, and Joseph Gusfield. Philadelphia: Temple University Press, 1994. 3–35.

Jones, L. R., and R. R. Parlour, eds. *Wyatt v. Stickney. Retrospect and Prospect*. New York: Grune and Stratton, 1981.

Jorgenson, Linda Mabus. Personal interview. 26 April 1995a.

———. "Sexual Contact in Fiduciary Relationships: Legal Perspectives." *Breach of Trust: Sexual Exploitation by Health Care Professionals and Clergy*. Ed. John C. Gonsiorek. Thousand Oaks, CA: Sage, 1995b. 237–83.

Jorgenson, Linda Mabus, Steven B. Bishing, and Pamela K. Sutherland. "Therapist–Patient Sexual Exploitation and Insurance Liability." *Tort and Insurance Law Journal* 27.3 (1992): 595–614.

Jorgenson, Linda Mabus, and Rebecca Randles. *Oklahoma Law Review* 44.2 (Summer 1991): 181–225.

Jorgenson, Linda, Rebecca Randles, and Larry Strasburger. "The Furor over Psychotherapist–Patient Sexual Contact: New Solutions to an Old Problem." *William and Mary Law Review* 32.3 (1991): 645–732.

Jorgenson, Linda Mabus, and Pamela K. Sutherland. "Fiduciary Theory Applied to Personal Dealings: Attorney–Client Sexual Contact." *Arkansas Law Review* 45.3 (1992): 459–503.

K. B. Personal communication. 16 May 1999.

Kahneman, D., and A. Tversky. "Prospect Theory: An Analysis of Decision under Risk." *Econometrica* 47 (March 1979): 263–91.

Kaminer, Wendy. *I'm Dysfunctional, You're Dysfunctional: The Recovery Movement and Other Self-Help Fashions*. Reading, MA: Addison-Wesley, 1992.

Kane, Andrew. "The Effects of Criminalization of Sexual Misconduct by Therapists: Report of a Survey in Wisconsin." *Breach of Trust: Sexual Exploitation by Health Care Professionals and Clergy*. Ed. John C. Gonsiorek. Thousand Oaks, CA: Sage, 1995. 317–33.

Karmen, Andrew. *Crime Victims: An Introduction to Victimology*. Pacific Grove, CA: Brooks/Cole, 1990.

Katz, A. H. *Self-Help in America: A Social Movement Perspective*. New York: Twayne, 1993.

Katz, A. H., H. L. Hedrick, D. H. Isenberg, L. M. Thompson, T. Goodrich, and A. H. Kutschner. *Self-Help. Concepts and Applications*. Philadelphia: Charles Press, 1992.

Keeton, W. Page, Dan B. Dobbs, Robert E. Keeton, and David G. Owen. *Prosser and Keeton on the Law of Torts*. St. Paul, MN: West, 1984.

Kingdon, John W. *Agendas, Alternatives, and Public Policies*. New York: Harper-Collins College, 1995.

Klandermans, Bert. "The Social Construction of Protest and Multiorganizational Fields." *Frontiers in Social Movement Theory*. Ed. Aldon D. Morris and Carol McClurg Mueller. New Haven, CT: Yale University Press, 1992. 77–103.

———. "Mobilization and Participation: Social Psychological Expansions of Resource Mobilization Theory." *American Sociological Review* 49 (1984): 583–600.

Klein, Ethel. "The Diffusion of Consciousness in the United States and Western Europe." *The Women's Movements of the United States and Western Europe: Consciousness, Political Opportunity, and Public Opinion*. Ed. Mary Fainsod and Carol McClurg Mueller. Philadelphia: Temple University Press, 1987. 23–43.

Koenig, Thomas, and Michael Rustard. "His and Her Tort Reform: Gender Injustice in Disguise." *Washington Law Review* 70.1 (1995): 1–90.

Koss, Mary P., and Mary R. Harvey. *The Rape Victim: Clinical and Community Interventions*. Newbury Park, CA: Sage, 1991.

Kuchan, Anthony. "Survey of Incidence of Psychotherapists' Sexual Contact with Clients in Wisconsin." *Psychotherapists' Sexual Involvement with Clients: Intervention and Prevention*. Ed. Gary Richard Schoener, Jeanette Hofstee Milgrom, John C. Gonsiorek, Ellen T. Luepker, and Ray M. Conroe. Minneapolis: Walk-In Counselling Center, 1989. 537–65.

Labaton, Stephen. "Are Divorce Lawyers Really the Sleaziest?" *New York Times* 5 September 1993: 5A.

Lacey, Nicola. *Unspeakable Subjects*. Oxford, England: Hart, 1998.

Langford, William D., Jr. "Criminalizing Attorney–Client Sexual Relations: Toward Substantive Enforcement." *Texas Law Review* 73 (1995): 1223–54.

Laverne. Personal interview. 15 October 1993.

Lazarus, Jeremy A. "Sex with Former Patients Almost Always Unethical." *American Journal of Psychiatry* 149 (1992): 855–57.

Lehr, Dick. "Psychiatrists and Sex Abuse: State Regulation Marked by Delay, Confusion, Loopholes." *Boston Globe* 4 October 1994: 1, 14.

Lewin, Tamar. "Tangled Case of Sexual Molestation Pits a Doctor Against 8 Poor Women." *New York Times* 29 January 1995, 20.

Lewis, Anthony. "Savaging the Great." *New York Times* 11 May 1994: A11.

Lewis, Laurel. "Growing beyond Abuse." *Breach of Trust: Sexual Exploitation by Health Care Professionals and Clergy*. Ed. John C. Gonsiorek. Thousand Oaks, CA: Sage, 1995. 49–51.

Linda. Personal communication. 21 April 1999.

Lindgren, J. Ralph, and Nadine Taub. *The Law of Sex Discrimination*. St. Paul, MN: West, 1994.

Lisa. Personal communication. 4 June 1999.

Lofland, John. *Deviance and Identity*. Englewood Cliffs, NJ: Prentice-Hall, 1969.

Loh, Wallace D. "Q: What Has Reform of Rape Legislation Wrought? A: Truth in Criminal Labelling." *Journal of Social Issues* 37 (1981): 28–52.

Luepker, Ellen. "Effects of Practitioners' Sexual Misconduct: A Follow-Up Study." *Journal of the American Academy of Psychiatry and the Law* (March 1999): 51–63.

———. "Helping Direct and Associate Victims to Restore Connections after Practitioner Sexual Misconduct." *Breach of Trust: Sexual Exploitation by Health Care Professionals and Clergy*. Ed. John C. Gonsiorek. Thousand Oaks, CA: Sage, 1995. 112–28.

———. Personal communication. 7 July 1993.

———. "Time-Limited Treatment/Support Groups for Clients Who Have Been Sexually Exploited by Therapists: A Nine Year Perspective." *Psychotherapists' Sexual Involvement with Clients: Intervention and Prevention*. Ed. Gary Richard Schoener, Jeanette Hofstee Milgrom, John C. Gonsiorek, Ellen T. Luepker, and Ray M. Conroe. Minneapolis: Walk-In Counselling Center, 1989. 181–94.

Luepker, Ellen Thompson, and Michael O'Brien. "Support Groups for Spouses." *Psychotherapists' Sexual Involvement with Clients: Intervention and Prevention*. Ed. Gary Richard Schoener, Jeanette Hofstee Milgrom, John C. Gonsiorek,

Ellen T. Luepker, and Ray M. Conroe. Minneapolis: Walk-In Counselling Center, 1989. 241–44.

Luepker, Ellen, and Carol Retsch-Bogart. "Group Treatment for Clients Who Have Been Sexually Involved with Their Psychotherapists." *Sexual Exploitation of Patients by Health Professionals.* Ed. Ann Burgess and Carol R. Hartmann. New York: Praeger, 1986. 163–72.

Maines, Rachel P. *The Technology of Orgasm: "Hysteria," the Vibrator, and Women's Sexual Satisfaction.* Baltimore: The Johns Hopkins University Press, 1999.

"Malpractice Crisis Largely Due to Few Doctors, Study Finds." *Gainesville Sun* 14 April 1986: 7A.

Marge. Personal interview. 25 June 1994.

Maris, Margo E., and Kevin M. McDonough. "How Churches Respond to the Victims and Offenders of Clergy Sexual Misconduct." *Breach of Trust: Sexual Exploitation by Health Care Professionals and Clergy.* Ed. John C. Gonsiorek. Thousand Oaks, CA: Sage, 1995. 348–67.

Marshall, Pat. "Auditing Institutions for the Tolerance of Sexual Misconduct: An Important Strategy for Dealing with Boundary Violations." Fourth International Conference, Boston, 3 October 1998.

Martz, E. Wayne. Personal communication. 21 April 1995.

Mary (Represenatative of Forbidden Zone Recovery Group). Personal interview. 3 November 1993.

Masters, William H., and Virginia E. Johnson. "Principles of the New Sex Therapy." *American Journal of Psychiatry* 133 (1976): 548–53.

———. "Principles of the New Sex Therapy." Paper delivered at the Annual Meeting of the American Psychiatric Association, Anaheim, CA 1975.

———. *Human Sexual Inadequacy.* Boston: Little, Brown, 1970.

Maton, K., G. Leventhal, E. Madara, and M. Julien. "Factors Affecting the Birth and Death of Mutual-Help Groups: The Role of National Affiliation, Professional Involvement, and Member Focal Problem." *American Journal of Community Psychology* 17.5 (1989): 643–71.

May, Marylynn L., and Daniel B. Stengel. "Who Sues Their Doctors? How Patients Handle Medical Grievances." *Law and Society Review* 24.1 (1990): 105–20.

McCarthy, John D. "Activists, Authorities, and Media Framing of Drunk Driving." *New Social Movements.* Ed. Hank Johnston, Enrique Larana, and Joseph Gusfield. Philadelphia: Temple University Press, 1994. 133–67.

McCartney, J. L. "Overt Transference." *Journal of Sex Research* 2 (1966): 227–37.

McLeod, Molly. Personal interview. 3 June 1994.

McNamara, Eileen. *Breakdown.* New York: Pocket Books, 1994.

Meyer, David S., and Joshua Gamson. "The Challenge of Cultural Elites: Celebrities and Social Movements." *Sociological Inquiry* 65.2 (1995): 181–206.

Meyer, David S., and Nancy Whittier. "Social Movement Spillover." *Social Problems* 41.2 (1994): 277–97.

Migliori, J. Personal interview. 27 October 1993.

Milgrom, Jeanette Hofstee. "Advocacy: Assisting Sexually Exploited Clients through the Complaint Process." *Psychotherapists' Sexual Involvement with Clients: Intervention and Prevention.* Ed. Gary Richard Schoener, Jeanette Hofstee Milgrom, John C. Gonsiorek, Ellen T. Luepker, and Ray M. Conroe. Minneapolis: Walk-In Counselling Center, 1989a. 305–12.

————. "Secondary Victims of Sexual Exploitation by Counselors and Therapists: Some Observations." *Psychotherapists' Sexual Involvement with Clients: Intervention and Prevention.* Ed. Gary Richard Schoener, Jeanette Hofstee Milgrom, John C. Gonsiorek, Ellen T. Luepker, and Ray M. Conroe. Minneapolis: Walk-In Counselling Center, 1989b. 235–40.

Minnesota Board of Medical Examiners. *Biennial Report.* St. Paul, MN, 1992.

Missing Link 5.2 (Summer / Fall 1997); 3.2 (Summer 1995); 3.1 (Spring 1995); 2.2 (Fall 1994).

Molloy, Bartholomew. Personal interview. 11 June 1993.

Mooney, Brian C. "The Patients Left Behind." *Boston Globe* 5 October 1994: 1, 18.

Morris, Aldon D. *The Origins of the Civil Rights Movement.* New York: Free Press, 1984.

Morris, Larry, and Garry Perrin. "Board Action—Sexual Intimacies with Patients." *The Arizona Psychologist* 14.3 (1994): 5.

Mueller, Carol McClurg. "Building Social Movement Theory." *Frontiers in Social Movement Theory.* New Haven, CT: Yale University Press, 1992. 3–25.

Murrell, Dan S., J. L. Bernard, Lisa K. Coleman, Deborah L. O'Laughlin, and Robert B. Gaia. "Loose Canons. A National Survey of Attorney–Client Sexual Involvement: Are There Ethical Concerns?" *Mississippi State University Law Review* 23.3 (1993): 483–506.

"My Doctor, My Lover." *Frontline.* PBS. 11 May 1993.

Nancy. Personal communication. 16 February 1999.

National Association of Social Workers Code of Ethics. Washington, DC: National Association of Social Workers, 1993.

Nelson, Barbara J. *Making an Issue Out of Child Abuse.* Chicago: University of Chicago Press, 1984.

News Release. Federation of State Boards of Medicine, Euless, TX, 25 March 1997.

Niebuhr, Gustav. "For a Cardinal and His Ex-Accuser, a Profound Reconciliation." *New York Times* 7 January 1994: 7.

Noel, Barbara, with Kathryn Watterson. *You Must Be Dreaming.* New York: Poseidon Press, 1992.

Noel, Margery. Personal communication. 29 May 1998.

Noel, Margery, and William E. Foote. "The Processes of Passing Criminal Legislation: The New Mexico Experience." It's Never O.K. Conference, Toronto, Canada, 14 October 1994.

Opp, Karl-Dieter. "Grievances and Participation in Social Movements." *American Sociological Review* 53 (December 1988): 853–64.

"Our Sleeping Doctor Watchers." *New York Times* 8 May 1995: 14.

Pagano, Phyllis J. "Heal Thyself: Therapy and the Betrayal of Trust." *The New Renaissance* 10.1 (1997a): 11–29.

————. Personal interview. 2 April 1997b; 9 June 1993.

PAN meeting, Los Angeles, 13 April 1996.

Park, Laurel. Personal interview. 15 October 1994.

Parker, Claudia. Personal interview. 20 March 1999; 3 April 1997.

Parsons, John P., and John P. Wincze. "A Survey of Client–Therapist Sexual Involvement in Rhode Island as Reported by Subsequent Treating Therapists." *Professional Psychology* 26.2 (1995): 171–75.

Paula. Personal communication. 2 February 1999.

Pavalon, Eugene I., and Thomas G. Alvary. "Protective and Secrecy Orders. Time for Change." *Trial* (March 1991): 110–14.

P. E. Personal interview. 17 May 1999.

"People v. Boyer." (97SA27) *National Law Journal* (21 April 1997): 20B.

Perr, Irvin. "Medicological Aspects of Professional Sexual Exploitation." *Sexual Exploitation in Professional Relationships*. Ed. Glen Gabbard. Washington, DC: American Psychiatric Press, 1989. 211–27.

Peterson, Marilyn R. *At Personal Risk: Boundary Violations in Professional–Client Relationships*. New York: W. W. Norton, 1992.

Peterson, Michael. "The Problem of Sexual Molestation by Roman Catholic Clergy: Meeting the Problem in a Comprehensive and Responsible Manner." Confidential document compiled for the National Conference of Catholic Bishops, 8–9 June 1985.

Phyllis. Personal interview. 9 June 1993.

Pitt, J. Personal interview. 29 October 1993.

Plaut, S. M., and B. H. Foster. "Role of the Health Professional in Cases Involving Sexual Exploitation of Patients." *Sexual Exploitation of Patients by Health Professionals*. Ed. Ann Burgess and Carol R. Hartman. New York: Praeger, 1986. 5–25.

Pogrebin, Mark R., Eric D. Poole, and Amos Martinez. "Accounts of Professional Misdeeds: The Sexual Exploitation of Clients by Psychotherapists." *Deviant Behavior: An Interdisciplinary Journal* 13 (1992): 229–52.

Pope, Kenneth, and Jacqueline Bouhoutsos. *Sexual Intimacy between Therapists and Patients*. Westport, CT: Praeger, 1986.

Pope, Kenneth S., and Melba J. T. Vasquez. *Ethics in Psychotherapy and Counselling*. San Francisco: Jossey-Bass, 1991.

Powell, T. J. *Working with Self-Help*. Silver Spring, MD: National Association of Social Workers, 1990.

———. *Self-Help Organizations and Professional Practice*. Silver Spring, MD: National Association of Social Workers, 1987.

"Priest Denies Targeting Cardinal." *Columbus Dispatch* 31 January 1997: 8A.

The Principles of Medical Ethics: With Annotations Especially Applicable to Psychiatry. Washington, DC: American Psychiatric Association, 1993.

Proclamations of Survivor Connections. Cranston, RI: Survivor Connections, n.d.

"Psychotherapy." *Newsweek* 13 April 1992.

Quadrio, Carolyn. "Sexual Abuse Involving Therapists, Clergy, and Judiciary: Closed Ranks, Collusions and Conspiracies of Silence." *Psychiatry, Psychology and Law* 1.2 (1994): 189–98.

Radlett-Kollar, Linda. PAN meeting, Los Angeles, 13 April 1996.

Reed, Kathleen. Personal interview. 9 August 1993.

"Report of the Ethics Committee." *American Psychologist* 49.7 (July 1994): 659–66.

Restoring the Integrity: Conference on the Dimensions of Sexual Exploitation by Professions Involved in Relationships of Trust, Fredericton, New Brunswick, Canada, 15–16 October 1993.

Rick. Personal interview. 8 November 1997.

Riger, Stephanie. "Gender Dilemmas in Sexual Harassment Policies and Procedures." *American Psychologist* 46.5 (May 1991): 497–505.

Roberts-Henry, Melissa. "Criminalization of Therapist Sex in Colorado: An Overview and Opinion." *Breach of Trust: Sexual Exploitation by Health Care Professionals and Clergy*. Ed. John C. Gonsiorek. Thousand Oaks, CA: Sage, 1995a. 338–47.

———. "Making the Leap: A Personal Story of Moving from Victim/Survivor to 'Activityist.'" *Breach of Trust: Sexual Exploitation by Health Care Professionals and Clergy*. Ed. John C. Gonsiorek. Thousand Oaks, CA: Sage, 1995b. 52–56.

Roberts, Melissa. Personal interview. 26 October 1995; 20 November 1993.

Roiphe, Katie. *The Morning After: Sex, Fear, and Feminism on Campus*. New York: Little, Brown, 1993.

Roney, John (Senator). Personal interview. 29 May 1998.

Roseman, Mark. "Recovery from Clergy Sexual Abuse: The Value of Social, Political and Legal Actions." Fourth International Conference, Boston, 3 October 1998.

Roseman, Mark. Personal interview. 8 February 1999; 9 November 1997.

Rosenberg, Gerald N. *The Hollow Hope*. Chicago: University of Chicago Press, 1991.

Rubino, Steven. Personal interview. 9 November 1997.

Russell, Sherry. Personal interview. 17 February 1999.

Rutter, Peter. *Sex in the Forbidden Zone: When Therapists, Doctors, Clergy, Teachers and Other Men in Power Betray Women's Trust*. Los Angeles: Jeremy P. Tarcher, 1989.

Sappington, Marlene. Personal interview. 12 February 1996.

Savage, Robert L. "When a Policy's Time Has Come: Cases of Rapid Policy Diffusions in 1983–4." *Publius* 15 (1985): 113–25.

Schechter, Susan. *Women and Male Violence*. Boston: South End Press, 1982.

Schiltz, Patrick. Personal interview. 23 June 1993.

Schmitt, Kara. *An Analysis of Complaints Filed against Mental Health Professionals in Colorado. Report for the Administrator of the Mental Health Professions*. Denver: Colorado Department of Regulatory Agencies, 1995.

Schoener, Gary Richard. Personal interviews: 1 March 1999; 19 May 1998; 21 February 1997; 21 October 1996; 19 April and 6 November 1995; 24 June 1993.

———. "Prevention and Intervention in Professional Misconduct: International Perspectives." Presentation to the Fourth International Conference on Sexual Misconduct by Psychotherapists, Other Health Care Professionals and Clergy. 30 October 1998.

———. "Identification and Prevention of Boundary Violations: Exercises and Tools." *Minnesota Psychologist* (7 March 1997): 7.

———. "Historical Overview." *Breach of Trust: Sexual Exploitation by Health Care Professionals and Clergy*. Ed. John C. Gonsiorek. Thousand Oaks, CA: Sage, 1995.

———. Presentation to It's Never O.K. Conference, 15 October 1994.

———. Personal communication. 21 April 1993a.

———. "Therapist–Client Sexual Involvement—Incidence and Prevalence." *Minnesota Psychologist* (January 1991): 14–15.

———. "Filing Complaints against Therapists Who Sexually Exploit Clients." *Psychotherapists' Sexual Involvement with Clients: Intervention and Prevention*.

Ed. Gary Richard Schoener, Jeanette Hofstee Milgrom, John C. Gonsiorek, Ellen T. Luepker, and Ray M. Conroe. Minneapolis: Walk-In Counselling Center, 1989a. 313–43.

———. "A Look at the Literature." *Psychotherapists' Sexual Involvement with Clients: Intervention and Prevention.* Ed. Gary Richard Schoener, Jeanette Hofstee Milgrom, John C. Gonsiorek, Ellen T. Luepker, and Ray M. Conroe. Minneapolis: Walk-In Counselling Center, 1989b. 11–50.

———. "Legislative Models for Dealing with Therapist/Patient Sex: Minnesota and Wisconsin." *Psychotherapists' Sexual Involvement with Clients: Intervention and Prevention.* Ed. Gary Richard Schoener, Jeanette Hofstee Milgrom, John C. Gonsiorek, Ellen T. Luepker, and Ray M. Conroe. Minneapolis: Walk-In Counselling Center, 1989c. 529–35.

———. "The New Laws." *Psychotherapists' Sexual Involvement with Clients: Intervention and Prevention.* Ed. Gary Richard Schoener, Jeanette Hofstee Milgrom, John C. Gonsiorek, Ellen T. Luepker, and Ray M. Conroe. Minneapolis: Walk-In Counselling Center, 1989d. 537–65.

Schoener, Gary Richard, Jeanette Hofstee Milgrom, John C. Gonsiorek, Ellen T. Luepker, and Ray M. Conroe. *Psychotherapists' Sexual Involvement with Clients: Intervention and Prevention.* Minneapolis: Walk-In Counselling Center, 1989.

Schuck, Peter H. "The New Juridical Ideology of Tort Law." *New Direction of Liability Law.* Ed. Walter Olson. New York: Academy of Political Science, 1988. 4–17.

Schulhofer, Stephen J. *Unwanted Sex: The Culture of Intimidation and the Failure of the Law.* Cambridge: Harvard University Press, 1998.

"Sex Abuse Bills in Limbo." *Boston Globe* 4 October 1994: 15.

"Sexual Exploitation: Strategies for Prevention and Intervention." *Report of the Maryland Task Force to Study Health Professional–Client Sexual Exploitation.* Maryland Department of Health and Mental Hygiene, 1996.

Sharon. Personal interview. 12 June 1993.

Shepard, Martin. *The Love Treatment: Sexual Intimacy between Patients and Psychotherapist.* New York: Peter H. Wyden, 1971.

Shiltz, Patrick. Personal interview. 25 June 1993.

Sloan, Lacey, Tonya Edmond, Allen Rubin, and Michael Doughty. "Social Workers' Knowledge of and Experiences with Sexual Exploitation by Psychotherapists." *Social Work* 43.1 (1998): 43–53.

SNAP (Survivors Network of Those Abused by Priests). First International SNAP Conference, Washington, DC, 8–10 November 1996.

Snow, David A., and Robert D. Benford. "Ideology, Frame Resonance, and Participant Mobilization." *International Social Movement Research.* Vol. 1: *From Structure to Action.* Ed. Bert Klandermans, Hanspeter Kriesi, and Sidney Tarrow. Greenwich, CT: JAI Press, 1988. 197–217.

———. "Master Frames and Cycles of Protest." *Frontiers in Social Movement Theory.* Ed. Aldon Morris and Carol M. Mueller. New Haven, CT: Yale University Press, 1992. 133–55.

Snow, David A., E. Burke Rochford, Jr., Steven K. Worden, and Robert D. Benford. "Frame Alignment Processes, Micromobilization, and Movement Participation." *American Sociological Review* 51 (August 1986): 464–81.

Spector, Malcolm, and John I. Kitsuse. *Constructing Social Problems*. New York: Aldine de Gruyter, 1977.

Spohn, Cassia, and Julie Horney. *Rape Law Reform: A Grass Roots Revolution and Its Impact*. New York: Plenum, 1992.

Starr, Paul. *The Social Transformation of American Medicine*. New York: Basic Books, 1982.

"State of Florida—Agency for Health Care Administration Memorandum to the Board of Medicine." *Subject 1994 Annual Disciplinary Report*. 20 January 1995.

Stedman's Medical Dictionary. Baltimore: Williams and Wilkins, 1990.

Steinberg, Lynn. Personal interview. 25 January 1999; 21 July 1997.

Steinfels, Peter. "$118 Million Damage Award for Sexual Abuse by Priest." *New York Times* 25 July 1997: 1A, 12A.

Survivor Activist 6.1 (Spring 1998); 5.2 (Autumn 1997); 5.1 (Spring 1997): Insert; 4.3 (Autumn 1996); 3.2 (Spring 1995); 3.1 (Winter 1995); 2.4 (Autumn 1994); 2.2 (Spring 1994).

Survivor Connections Introductory Package. Cranston, RI: Survivor Connections, n.d.

Swidler, Ann. "Culture in Action: Symbols and Strategies." *American Sociological Review* 51.2 (1986): 273–86.

Tarrow, Sidney. *Power in Movement: Social Movements, Collective Action and Mass Politics in the Modern State*. Cambridge: Cambridge University Press, 1994.

Task Force on Sexual Abuse of Patients: Report. Ontario: College of Physicians and Surgeons of Ontario, Canada, 1991.

Taylor, Verta. *Rock-a-By-Baby: Feminism, Self-Help and Post-Partum Depression*. New York: Routledge, 1996.

Taylor, Verta, and Nancy Whittier. "Analytical Approaches to Social Movement Culture: The Culture of the Women's Movement." *Social Movements and Culture*. Eds. Hank Johnston and Bert Klandermans. Minneapolis: University of Minnesota Press, 1995. 163–87.

TELL Starterkit. Waban, MA, 1993.

Terry. Personal interview. 13 May 1993.

To Tell the Truth. Conference organized by Survivor Connections, Providence, RI, 1 October 1994.

Tong, Rosemarie. *Women, Sex, and the Law*. Totawa, NJ: Rowman and Allanheld, 1984.

Urquhart, Lynne. Personal interview. 12 April 1999.

Van Voris, Bob. "Mormons Hit by Child–Sex Lawsuits." *National Law Journal* (16 November 1998): 1A.

Vinson, Jane S. "Use of Complaint Procedures in Cases of Therapist–Patient Sexual Contact." *Professional Psychology: Research and Practice* 18.2 (1987): 159–64.

———. *Sexual Contact with Psychotherapists: A Study of Client Reactions and Complaint Procedures*. Berkeley: California School of Professional Psychology, 1984.

Walker, Evelyn, and Perry Dean Young. *A Killing Cure*. New York: Henry Holt, 1986.

Weaver, Dianne Jay. "Secrets That Can Kill Have No Place in Our Courts." *Product Safety and Liability Reporter*. Washington, DC: Bureau of National Affairs. (15 June 1991): 701–5.

Weed, Frank J. "The Victim–Activist Role in the Anti-Drunk Driving Movement." *Sociological Quarterly* 31.3 (1990): 459–73.

Whitfield, Charles. "Memory and Abuse." Presentation at the Linkup Conference, 8 November 1997.

Winn, James R. "Medical Boards and Sexual Misconduct: An Overview of Federation Data." *Federation Bulletin* (Summer 1993): 88–92.

Wisc. Stat. Ann. s.940.22(2) (West Supp. 1990).

Wohlberg, Jan W. "Ethics' Committees: The Good, the Bad, and the Ugly." Presentation to the Fourth International Conference on Sexual Misconduct by Psychotherapists, Other Health Care Professionals and Clergy, 3 October 1998.

————. Personal interview. 5 September 1995; 16 October 1993.

————. "Sexual Abuse in the Therapeutic Setting: What Do Victims Really Want?" Presented to Boston Psychoanalytic Society and Institute's Symposium on New Psychoanalytic Perspectives on the Treatment of Sexual Abuse, Boston, 1994.

————. "Healing from Within: Role of Support Groups." Restoring the Integrity Conference, Fredericton, New Brunswick, Canada, 1993.

Wollert, R., N. Barron, and M. Bob. "Parents United of Oregon: A Natural History of a Self-Help Group for Sexually Abusive Families." *Prevention in Human Services* 1.3 (1982): 99–109.

Yaukey, B. Personal interview. 25 October 1993.

Zelen, Seymour L. "Sexualization of Therapeutic Relationships: The Dual Vulnerability of Patient and Therapist." *Psychotherapy* 22.2 (1985): 178–85.

INDEX